Women's Edge
HEALTH ENHANCEMENT GUIDE™

# Natural Remedies

## *Nondrug Healing Strategies That Work Best*

By the Editors of

*PREVENTION*
Health Books
*for* Women™

RODALE

© 1999 by Rodale Inc.
Illustrations © 1999 by Shawn Banner, Narda Lebo, Tom Ward

All rights reserved. No part of this publication may be reproduced or transmitted in any form or by any means, electronic or mechanical, including photocopying, recording, or any other information storage and retrieval system, without the written permission of the publisher.

*Prevention* Health Books for Women and Women's Edge Health Enhancement Guide are trademarks of Rodale Inc.

Printed in the United States of America on acid-free ∞, recycled paper ♻

**Library of Congress Cataloging-in-Publication Data**

Natural remedies : nondrug healing strategies that work best / by the
    editors of Prevention Health Books for Women.
       p.   cm. — (Women's edge health enhancement guide)
     ISBN 1–57954–103–8 hardcover
     1. Women—Health and hygiene.  2. Naturopathy.  3. Self-care,
Health.  4. Medicine, Popular.   I. Prevention Health Books for
Women.  II. Series.
RA778.N384   1999
613'.04244—dc21                           99–19847

**Distributed to the book trade by St. Martin's Press**

  4  6  8  10  9  7  5  3     hardcover

Visit us on the Web at www.rodalebooks.com, or call us toll-free at (800) 848-4735.

WE **INSPIRE** AND **ENABLE** PEOPLE TO IMPROVE
THEIR LIVES AND THE WORLD AROUND THEM

**EDITOR:** Debora T. Yost

**SERIES EDITOR:** E. A. Tremblay

**STAFF WRITERS:** Susan G. Berg, Bridget Doherty, Arden Moore

**CONTRIBUTING WRITERS:** Leah Flickinger, Grete Haentjens, Sarí Harrar, Lois Guarino Hazel, Jennifer L. Kaas, Mary Kittel, Nanci Kulig, Sandra Salera Lloyd, Gale Maleskey, Holly McCord, Deanna Moyer, Sara Altshul O'Donnell, Deborah Pedron, Kathryn Piff, Judith Springer Riddle, Carla Thomas, Julia VanTine, Shea Zukowski

**ART DIRECTOR:** Darlene Schneck

**SERIES ART DIRECTOR:** Diane Ness Shaw

**SERIES DESIGNER:** Lynn N. Gano

**COVER AND INTERIOR DESIGNER:** Diane Ness Shaw

**ILLUSTRATORS:** Shawn Banner, Narda Lebo, Diane Ness Shaw, Tom Ward

**ASSOCIATE RESEARCH MANAGER:** Anita C. Small

**BOOK PROJECT RESEARCHER:** Shea Zukowski

**EDITORIAL RESEARCHERS:** Molly Donaldson Brown, Lori Davis, Adrien Drozdowksi, Leah Flickinger, Carol J. Gilmore, Bella Hebrew, Karen Jacob, Jennifer L. Kaas, Mary S. Mesaros, Paris Muchanic, Elizabeth Price, Paula Rasich, Staci Ann Sander, Amy Seirer, Lucille S. Uhlman

**SENIOR COPY EDITORS:** Amy K. Kovalski, Karen Neely

**PRODUCTION EDITOR:** Cindy Updegrove

**LAYOUT DESIGNER:** Donna G. Rossi

**ASSOCIATE STUDIO MANAGER:** Thomas P. Aczel

**MANUFACTURING COORDINATORS:** Brenda Miller, Jodi Schaffer, Patrick T. Smith

## Rodale Healthy Living Books

VICE PRESIDENT AND PUBLISHER: Brian Carnahan

VICE PRESIDENT AND EDITORIAL DIRECTOR: Debora T. Yost

VICE PRESIDENT AND MARKETING DIRECTOR: Karen Arbegast

EDITORIAL DIRECTOR: Michael Ward

WRITING DIRECTOR: Brian Paul Kaufman

PRODUCT MARKETING MANAGER: Guy Maake

BOOK MANUFACTURING DIRECTOR: Helen Clogston

MANUFACTURING MANAGERS: Eileen Bauder, Mark Krahforst

RESEARCH MANAGER: Ann Gossy Yermish

COPY MANAGER: Lisa D. Andruscavage

PRODUCTION MANAGER: Robert V. Anderson Jr.

OFFICE MANAGER: Roberta Mulliner

OFFICE STAFF: Jacqueline Dornblaser, Julie Kehs, Suzanne Lynch, Mary Lou Stephen

# The New Age of Healing

Want to be on the forefront of the twenty-first century health revolution?

Then bone up on the natural remedies in this book—and start taking charge of your own health.

The 1990s have seen American women embrace natural healing in astounding numbers. Since 1990, use of herbal remedies in the United States has increased 380 percent, and use of vitamins for healing has risen 130 percent—figures, by the way, that come from that bastion of traditionalism and mainstream medical practice, the *Journal of the American Medical Association*. Their beliefs were once the antithesis of natural healing.

But things are changing.

Today, the majority of U.S. medical schools offers courses in alternative medicine. And more and more highly regarded medical centers, such as the University of Pennsylvania Medical Center in Philadelphia and Beth Israel Medical Center in New York City, are opening integrated medicine centers where treatments will combine alternative and traditional approaches.

All that is good news, but our own research here at *Prevention* Health Books shows another trend that is even more interesting: Women prefer to treat themselves. That's why they find natural remedies so appealing.

The natural therapies that women are using more often include herbs, vitamins, folk remedies, homeopathy, massage, and self-help groups. They most frequently use them to treat chronic conditions, such as back problems, headaches, depression, and anxiety.

If you're among the increasing number of women interested in exploring the world of natural healing, this volume of the Women's Edge health series belongs in your medicine chest. The information you'll find in this book was culled from interviews with more than 100 of the nation's leading practitioners of natural healing. Every piece of advice was checked by our own staff of researchers to ensure its accuracy and your safety.

Even natural medicine can have side effects, so please read the precautions in the Safe Use Guidelines chart on page 176 before treating yourself. And if you're pregnant or under medical care for any problem, it's a good idea to check with your doctor before taking any natural supplements.

Here's to natural *and* safe healing.

*Anne Alexander*

Anne Alexander
Editor-in-Chief, *Prevention* Magazine

# Contents

# PART ONE

# Feel Your Best

# Soothe Everyday Annoyances

**H**eadaches. Backaches. Hives. A lot of us can't seem to get through a day, let alone a week, without some minor health nuisance interfering with our lives. But consider yourself lucky. There are dozens of easy ways to solve life's little health glitches.

"Many health problems common to women respond very well to self-care," says Jill Stansbury, N.D., assistant professor of botanical medicine at the National College of Naturopathic Medicine in Portland, Oregon, and a naturopathic physician in Battle Ground, Washington. And many of the most successful self-care techniques are home remedies that have existed for decades, passed down through generations of caregivers.

Got a cold? Sure, the modern home remedy—cough syrup—works just fine. But you might find out that the century-old technique of drinking marsh mallow tea works even better.

And there's no doubt that over-the-counter antihistamines can do wonders for the itching of hives. But if you want to bypass drugs altogether, try what your great-great-grandmother probably did—soak in an oatmeal bath.

To find the best remedies for women's minor health problems, we interviewed caregivers and doctors for successful solutions to the most vexing little health problems. Here are the top picks for solving women's everyday annoyances.

## Aches and Pains

Most sudden (what doctors call acute) pain involves muscles—particularly muscles that are weak, tense, or in spasm. They crowd and irritate neighboring nerves, which registers as discomfort or dull pain somewhere in your body.

It may sound contradictory, but you can often avoid pain simply by making those muscles work harder. Research into sports medicine has shown that stretching and movement helps keep muscles flexible. And it not only benefits the muscles but the joints that they serve as well. Muscles that are flexible increase the range of motion of the nearby joints. This improves the flow of synovial fluid, the joint's lubricant, which nourishes the joint and reduces or prevents pain—much like the flow of oil keeps an engine running smoothly.

But even the best-oiled machine needs some tinkering from time to time. So when you get that ache-all-over feeling, here's what to do.

**Add ginger to your bath.** Sprinkle two tablespoons of powdered ginger into a tub of warm water, then climb in for a 20-minute soak. The ginger-water combination creates a sensation of heat, which helps relieve pain.

**Gently stretch away soreness.** Yoga, with its gentle stretching movements, can help ease and even prevent most body aches. Practice the following sequence.

❧ Stand with your arms over your head and your feet shoulder-width apart. Bend to the left, exhaling as you do. Hold for three seconds, then inhale as you return to an upright position. Do the same to the right side. Repeat three or four times, alternately bending left and right.

❧ Still standing with your feet shoulder-width apart, place your hands on your lower back and lift your chest. Gently bend backward, inhaling as you do. Hold for a few seconds, then return to an upright position. Exhale on your way back up. Repeat three times.

❧ Stand with your hands on your lower back and your feet shoulder-width apart. Bend your knees slightly and lean forward as far as is comfortable, exhaling as you do. Hold for three seconds, then return to an upright position, inhaling as you straighten up. Repeat three times.

---

## THE 10 BEST HICCUP CURES

When you least expect it, a nasty little nerve impulse tells your diaphragm to spasm, creating a chain reaction that makes your voice box close up, and *hic*—you have the hiccups.

To get rid of hiccups, you have to short-circuit the network that is making your diaphragm bounce about so annoyingly, explains Melissa Palmer, M.D., a gastroenterologist in Plainview, New York.

Of course, we all know this is easier said than done. There are enough home remedies for hiccups to fill an entire book, some of which would make you look and feel mighty foolish. One woman told us a case of stubborn hiccups went away instantly when a male colleague she barely knew jumped up, leaned across the meeting-room table, and kissed her squarely on the lips!

But you don't have to resort to such drastic measures. We took a poll on the most dependable hiccup remedies and came up with this Top 10 List.

1. Place a spoonful of granulated sugar under your tongue and let it dissolve.
2. Gently rub the back of your throat with a soft swab.
3. Pull on your tongue.
4. Put a little ice on the skin around the front of your throat just above your collarbone.
5. Chew papaya digestive tablets (available at health food stores) or a slice of fresh papaya or pineapple.
6. Make yourself sneeze by sniffing a dash of pepper.
7. Slowly sip a glass of ice water.
8. Hold your breath for 30 seconds.
9. Breathe in and out of a paper bag.
10. Pull your knees into your chest and lean forward to decrease pressure on your diaphragm.

---

**Chill it out.** For muscle strain that is painful but not debilitating, apply ice wrapped in a towel to the affected area. Leave the ice in place for 20 minutes for large muscles (such as those in the back), 10 to 15 minutes for small muscles (such as those in the elbows and calves), and 5 minutes for painful muscles in the face, hands, or feet. Repeat six times a day—three of those times in the evening—until the pain is reduced by half.

## Bad Breath

Bad breath is another universal complaint. Fiery and odorous foods, such as garlic, are obvious causes. Not so obvious: *not* eating. If you avoid mouthwatering meals, you may naturally decrease the amount of saliva that fights odor-causing bacteria in your mouth. Some women find that their breath seems more malodorous around the time of their periods. Bad breath can also be the sign of upcoming gum disease.

Popping a breath mint or swishing mouthwash masks the problem but doesn't eliminate it. The following remedies will freshen your breath naturally.

**Have an after-dinner drink of water.** Simply swishing a mouthful of water around your mouth after eating can deter bad breath. As a bonus, it helps wash away plaque, the sticky buildup of bacteria and tartar that leads to tooth decay and gum disease.

**Go for the garnish.** That sprig of parsley you find on the diner's blue plate special has a history and a purpose. A few nibbles are enough to vanquish stale breath. Parsley is a rich source of chlorophyll, which is a powerful breath freshener. If you don't like the taste, try parsley capsules instead. They're available in drugstores and some supermarkets.

**Sip a cup of tea.** Brew four whole cloves and two tablespoons of crumbled-up cinnamon sticks in one quart of water. Bring to a boil, cover, and simmer for 5 minutes. Remove the pot from the heat and let the tea steep for 20 minutes. Strain, allow to cool, and drink. Both cloves and cinnamon are potent antiseptics that can dissipate bad breath.

## Belching

A belch is nothing more than air making an explosive exit from your body. Once a belch passes your lips, there's little you can do except blush and say, "Excuse me." You're better off trying to prevent them in the first place. Here's how.

**Eat something.** When your stomach becomes too empty, it fills up with gassy air. Eventually, that air has to go someplace—namely, out. You can easily avoid this by not skipping meals.

**Chew, chew, chew.** Eating fast and gulping your food causes you to swallow a lot of air. Take your time and chew your food thoroughly.

**Hang loose.** Tight-fitting garments force air up and out of your digestive tract. Stick with loose, comfortable clothing.

## Blisters

As painful as a blister can be, it serves a very important purpose. It acts as a natural bandage, protecting the wound underneath from infection. And the fluid inside keeps the skin moist, so the wound heals quickly.

Blisters on the hands usually result from the friction generated during activities like raking and sweeping. In most cases, they're best left intact, but sometimes they're so large and uncomfortable that popping them is the only way to provide relief. Or they may open on their own.

With that in mind, here are the basics of blister care that you can use wherever blisters appear.

**Pop properly.** If you decide to pop a blister, first sterilize a needle with the flame of a match or rubbing alcohol. Then prick the "bubble" at the lowest point on your body. That way, gravity helps to drain the fluid and relieve pressure.

**Save your skin.** Whether you pop a blister or it breaks open on its own, leave that little flap of skin in place. It provides protection for the wound underneath.

**Keep it clean.** Gently wash the blister with soap and water. Use liquid soap if it's available. Bar soap may be coated with bacteria from previous uses.

**Wrap it up.** Once you have cleaned the blister, cover it with a bandage. This not only keeps out dirt and germs but also provides a comfortable cushion against friction. If your blister is open, coat it with a first-aid antibiotic ointment such as Mycitracin or Polysporin before applying the bandage. (Pure aloe vera gel can also help heal blisters because it contains both anti-inflammatory and antibiotic properties. It is sold in drugstores.)

## Bloating

One of two things are to blame for bloating—water or air. During your menstrual cycle, your body's supply of the hormone progesterone drops off in the 7 to 10 days before your period. Your body responds by storing salt, which in turn leads to water retention.

But bloating can also result from air that's either swallowed when you eat or produced in your digestive tract by high-fiber foods.

Here's what you can do.

**Step out for a stroll.** Walking or other light exercise can work wonders for bloating. It dispels gas and alleviates that feeling of distension.

**Drink dandelion tea.** For premenstrual bloating, dandelion tea helps the body eliminate excess water. To make the tea, add one teaspoon of dandelion (either the root or the whole herb) to one cup of boiling water. Let steep for five minutes, then strain and allow to cool. Drink a cup of the tea two or three times a day.

---

### WOMEN ASK WHY

*Why do paper cuts hurt so darn much?*

Paper delivers razor-sharp pain because paper has razor-sharp edges. To compound the problem, your fingertips, the usual targets for paper cuts, have the highest density of nerve endings of any part of your body.

So what do you do when you get a paper cut? Rinse it immediately under warm water to wash away the germs. Then clean it with hydrogen peroxide. Seal and protect it with petroleum jelly or an antibacterial salve. Then cover it with a bandage or waterproof first-aid tape to keep it closed and speed healing. Or you can dab it with a superglue. (It might sting a little, but it's safe.)

To avoid reliving the pain, don't try slicing any lemons. Getting anything acidic on a paper cut can be very painful. The same goes for skin-care products like hand lotions or creams that contain fragrances and preservative chemicals. These can sting when applied to open skin.

*Expert consulted*
*Debra Jaliman, M.D.*
*Clinical instructor of dermatology*
*Mt. Sinai Medical Center*
*New York City*

---

*Note:* Women who are taking diuretics—for high blood pressure, for example—should not drink dandelion tea. And if you have gallbladder disease, you should not use dandelion without your doctor's okay.

**Just add water.** Surprise! Consuming more liquids can actually reduce premenstrual bloating by diluting sodium in the body. Aim for a minimum of eight eight-ounce glasses of water a day.

**Choose foods carefully.** Certain foods produce a lot of gas and, therefore, contribute to bloating. Be wary of raw vegetables, cabbage, beans, and bagels and pretzels (both of which are cooked in boiling, bubbly water).

## Body Odor

Sweat has no odor, but it provides a moist breeding ground for bacteria. These bacteria eventually mix with a milky secretion from the apocrine glands, which are concentrated in the hairy areas under the arms and around the genitals. It's this brew that's responsible for body odor.

Most women can control body odor with a daily shower and deodorant. For those times when you need a little extra artillery, these strategies can help.

**Lather up.** Remember, body odor occurs only when bacteria mixes with the secretion from the apocrine glands. So you can minimize odor by using an antibacterial soap to cleanse the areas where the apocrine glands are concentrated—namely, under the arms and around the genitals. Once a day should do it.

**Buy the right deodorant.** For your underarms, choose an antiperspirant/deodorant combination that has aluminum chlorhydrate as its active ingredient. Such products minimize moisture, so bacteria have no place to grow.

**Add cornstarch.** Applying cornstarch to odor-prone areas also minimizes moisture, which discourages bacterial growth. (Avoid using baby powder or talcum powder because use of these products in the genital area has been linked to ovarian cancer.)

## Canker Sores

These craterlike sores—yellow at the base and red at the edges—can show up almost anywhere inside your mouth. No one knows for certain what causes them or why some people get them and others don't. For many women, stress and the menstrual cycle seem to be factors.

Left untreated, a canker sore usually goes away on its own in about two weeks. In the meantime, it can make routine activities such as talking and eating difficult and painful. To speed up the healing process, heed this advice.

**Try a little Tea-L-C.** Tannin, a compound in tea, seems to reduce the pain associated with canker sores. Soak a regular tea bag in warm water for a few minutes. Then squeeze out the excess water and place the tea bag directly on the canker sore for about five minutes. Repeat two or three times a day.

**Watch what you eat.** Certain fruits and vegetables—especially citrus fruits—are highly acidic, which can make a canker sore hurt more.

Spicy foods can also aggravate pain. And some nuts, especially walnuts, can trigger an allergic response that leads to a canker sore.

**Consider unexpected sources.** Many women get canker sores as an allergic response to chewing gum, mouthwashes, menthol cigarettes, lozenges, and common medications such as aspirin and ibuprofen. If you seem to get a canker sore every time you put a certain something in your mouth, you're better off avoiding it.

## Dry Mouth

Older women who are taking medications often experience dry mouth. But the condition can affect any woman at any age, for any number of reasons.

For instance, you can get dry mouth simply by breathing through your mouth rather than your nose—such as when you're congested or under stress. More seriously, dry mouth can be a symptom of Sjögren's syndrome, an autoimmune disease that strikes women much more frequently than men. In addition, women who have diabetes are at increased risk for dry mouth, as are women who have undergone radiation therapy for head and neck cancer.

Combating dry mouth requires a two-pronged approach. First, you want to stimulate your salivary glands to put out as much "juice" as possible. Second, you want to compensate for any saliva shortfall. Here's what you need to do.

**Get your jaw going.** Chewing sugarless gum jump-starts saliva production while moistening the inside of your mouth. If you're not a gum fan, any chewy food will do.

**Pick up a lemon drop.** Sucking on a sugarless lemon drop activates the salivary glands. Or, if you prefer, squeeze lemon into a glass of water, then drink up.

**Stay wet with water.** Carry a water bottle with you and sip every 10 minutes or so. The water helps keep your mouth moist and fresh.

Steer clear of soft drinks and fruit juices, though. Without saliva to neutralize it, the sugar in these drinks can really do a number on your teeth.

**Practice good dental hygiene.** Because dry mouth encourages cavity formation, you need to brush and floss regularly to keep your teeth healthy.

## Fever

A fever is not a disease. Rather, it's your body's way of protecting itself against invasive organisms, such as viruses and bacteria.

When you pick up a flu virus, for example, your immune system alerts your brain that it needs more heat in order to combat the virus. In response, your body temperature rises.

Truth be told, doctors don't agree on whether a fever requires treatment. The best advice: If it goes over 104°F, see your doctor right away. If it's under 104°F and making you miserable, by all means take steps to make yourself comfortable until your fever breaks. Here's what to do.

**Make a splash.** If you're hot and perspiring, draw a lukewarm bath and step in for a soak. Make sure the water is lukewarm, not cold. You don't want to get the chills.

**Stay hydrated.** As you perspire, you lose a lot of water. So be sure to keep your fluid intake up. Water is best, but fruit juices also help.

**Get some rest.** No playing superwoman! Your body demands rest while you have a fever. So stay in bed until your fever has been broken for at least 24 hours. Ask family and friends to pitch in with the cooking and laundry.

## Flatulence

If flatulence weren't so downright embarrassing, we might be able to appreciate just how common it is. The average woman passes gas 12 times a day, the same as the average man.

Gender doesn't influence flatulence much, but

eating habits certainly do. Ironically, many of the foods that are the most nutritious also produce the most gas: beans, broccoli, brussels sprouts, cabbage, cauliflower, corn, eggplant, garlic, onions, and radishes.

If the pressure builds, passing gas can be painful. But usually the discomfort is more social than physical. To put a stop to the sputtering, try these fast-acting tips.

**Check out charcoal.** Activated charcoal absorbs whatever is in your intestines, including gas and food particles that might later be turned into gas. Look for it in drugstores and follow the label instructions for dosage.

**Chew fennel seeds.** Fennel helps to dissipate gas by relaxing muscle spasms in the digestive tract. Chewing one-half teaspoon of seeds is usually enough to leave you flatulence-free.

**Pull the plug on pressure.** To alleviate gas pressure in your lower abdomen, try this simple exercise. Lie on your back with your knees bent. Then alternately raise each knee toward your chest until you feel relief.

**Break out the Beano.** Among foods, beans have a reputation as the most potent gas-producers around. You can render them gasless with a sprinkle of Beano. This liquid enzyme breaks down the indigestible sugars in beans. You can buy Beano in drugstores.

## Hives

Hives are small, red, intensely itchy bumps that appear alone or in clusters on the surface of the skin. They occur when something causes cells to release an inflammatory substance called histamine.

That "something" could be just about anything, from food to medication to stress. Even intense exercise or a hot shower can produce the dreaded tiny welts in people prone to them.

Hives usually go away on their own within a few hours. (If they don't, see a doctor.) In the meantime, these self-care measures can help stop the itch.

**Apply ice.** Rubbing an ice cube over the affected area for several minutes can actually help shrink the hives. Keep the cube moving, so it doesn't freeze the surface of your skin.

*Note:* This remedy is not appropriate for anyone who develops hives when exposed to cold.

**Sit in some oatmeal.** Colloidal oatmeal effectively relieves the itching associated with hives. Following the package instructions, add the powder to a tub of lukewarm water, then climb in and soak for 10 to 15 minutes. Make sure that the water is lukewarm. Hot water can aggravate hives.

**Stay cool, hang loose.** Because heat can make hives worse, try to keep yourself as cool as possible. You'll also feel more comfortable if you wear loose-fitting clothes.

**Pop a quercetin pill.** If you get hives when you eat certain foods, try taking 250 milligrams of quercetin 20 minutes before eating them. A plant compound, quercetin has antihistamine properties, which may discourage outbreaks. Quercetin supplements are sold in health food stores and some drugstores, often in combination with vitamin C.

## Muscle Cramps

A muscle cramp is your body's way of telling you that you have an imbalance of electrolytes. These substances keep cells functioning efficiently. The imbalance occurs when you don't have enough fluid in your system.

You can get a muscle cramp after exercising or overexerting yourself and from not drinking enough fluid. When that happens, the muscles tighten and shorten.

A muscle cramp can also strike when muscles are fatigued from overwork. These cramps often occur hours after an activity—while you're sitting or lying down, for example.

With a little coaxing, a muscle cramp will usually uncramp itself in no time. Follow this advice.

**Let your fingers do the working.** When you get a cramp, your first instinct may be to rub the affected area. And that's exactly what you should do. Gently massage the muscle until it relaxes.

**Make nice with ice.** Ice relieves pain and reduces inflammation. Try rubbing an ice cube over the affected area for two to three minutes. Or wrap an ice pack in a towel and lay it on the sore muscle for 20 minutes.

**Turn up the heat.** For some people, heat works better than ice in relieving a muscle cramp. Apply a heating pad for 20 minutes. If you don't have one, take a warm bath or shower instead.

**Drink up.** If you routinely get muscle cramps when you're active, chances are that you're not keeping yourself adequately hydrated. Remember to consume fluids before, during, and after any activity.

## Sore Throat

We usually interpret a sore throat as a sure sign of an impending cold. Yet as often as not, something else is to blame. Dry air, dust, tobacco smoke, and misdirected stomach acid can dry out the mucous membrane that lines the respiratory airways. Even a marathon session of talking or cheering can leave throat tissues painfully raw and irritated.

With time and a little TLC, a sore throat usually gets better on its own. If your throat is

### CRAMP, CRAMP GO AWAY

It grabs you like an invisible vise, squeezing your muscle with amazing speed and making you buckle in pain. But coiling in pain will only prolong it. The quickest way to get rid of a cramp is to gently stretch the muscle out. For a cramp in the leg, try these stretches, says Rosemary Agostini, M.D., clinical associate professor of orthopedics at the University of Washington and staff physician at the Virginia Mason Sports Medicine Center, both in Seattle.

**For a cramp in your calf, stand an arm's length (two to three feet) away from a wall. Bend the knee of the noncramped leg and step back with the other leg about two feet. Be sure to keep your back leg straight and both feet flat on the floor. Place your hands on the wall and bring your hips toward the wall while keeping your neck in line with your spine. Hold for 30 seconds, then stand up.**
**After stretching out, massage or ice the affected area.**

**For a cramp in your hamstring (at the back of your thigh), sit on the floor with your cramped leg straight out in front of you. Bend your noncramped leg so that your foot is next to the knee of your cramped leg. Lean forward from your waist until you feel a stretch in the back of the thigh of the cramped leg. Hold for 20 to 30 seconds, then relax.**

extremely painful and you're having difficulty swallowing, see your doctor. You may have strep throat, which requires medical attention. To help ease the pain, try the following strategies.

## FOLK REMEDY: DOES IT WORK?

### Honey for a Sore Throat

There's a good reason why Grandma would stir honey into a cup of steaming tea whenever her throat was feeling scratchy—honey kills bacteria.

"Honey is active against a wide range of bacterial and fungal species, many of which cause infections," says Angela Stengler, N.D., a naturopathic physician in Oceanside, California.

Honey's reputation as a folk cure for almost every ailment is exaggerated, however, Dr. Stengler notes. "Honey's antimicrobial effects would be so diluted after you swallow it that the honey probably couldn't kill bacteria throughout your whole body."

Yet honey is strong enough to kill some bacteria in your throat or at least soothe inflamed tissue there. Try stirring a teaspoon of it into a cup of hot tea or hot lemonade.

This remedy is safe for everyone except babies under one year of age. Honey contains dormant spores that are harmless to children and adults but may cause botulism in infants.

**RECOMMENDATION:** Worth a Try

jar. Let the herb steep overnight. The next morning, strain the tea and add four teaspoons of honey. Sip one-quarter to one-half cup of tea at a time over the course of the day.

*Note:* Marsh mallow may slow the absorption of other medications taken at the same time.

**Consider zinc.** At the first sign of a sore throat, begin sucking on zinc gluconate lozenges. The tablets work best if you place them on your tongue and allow them to dissolve. These lozenges bathe throat tissues in a soothing zinc solution. You can buy zinc gluconate lozenges at health food stores and drugstores.

**Avoid post-supper snoozing.** Lying down too soon after a meal allows stomach acid to back up into your throat. The acid burns delicate throat tissues. This is one reason why you should eat your dinner no less than four hours before bedtime.

## Tension Headache

By one estimate, almost everyone in the United States—approximately 90 percent of the population—has experienced a tension headache. This is no big surprise, considering that headaches are usually a by-product of stress.

But stress is not the only cause. In fact, everything from blocked sinuses to skipped meals can also trigger a tensionlike headache. In women, hormonal changes associated with menstruation or menopause are sometimes responsible.

A tension headache usually begins in the muscles at the back of your neck and slowly creeps toward your forehead. It may cause a throbbing sensation in your temples or behind your eyes.

**Grab the saltshaker.** Gargling with warm salt water gently cleanses a sore throat and helps draw fluid from inflamed tissues. To make a saltwater rinse, mix one-half teaspoon of salt with one cup of warm water. Spit out the salt water when you're finished. Repeat four or five times a day.

**Mend with marsh mallow.** No, not the sticky sweet stuff. Marsh mallow is an herb that quiets coughs and moistens and soothes a sore throat. To make a tea, place one-quarter cup of dried, chopped herb (sold in health food stores) in a glass or ceramic jar. Pour one pint of room-temperature water over the herb, then close the

Untreated, a tension headache usually subsides within a few hours. While an over-the-counter pain reliever can speed up the process, you may find that some of these natural remedies work just as well.

**Draw the pain out with water.** At the first sign of a tension headache, head for the nearest sink. Adjust the water temperature so that it's comfortably hot, then run your hands and wrists under the water for about 10 minutes. The heat draws blood away from your head and down into your hands, which may help relieve the pain.

**Sniff a soothing scent.** Keep a bottle of peppermint essential oil (available at health food stores and bath-and-beauty shops) on hand. Then take a whiff straight from the bottle whenever a tension headache has you in its grip. The smell of peppermint short-circuits headache pain fast by improving circulation and drawing energy away from the pain.

**Target your temples.** Position your thumbs on either side of your head, right in the center of each temple. Using a firm, circular motion, massage your temples for a minute or two.

**Schedule some tub time.** Steep two tablespoons of lavender and two tablespoons of lemon balm in one cup of hot water for 10 minutes. Pour the tea into a tub filled with lukewarm water, then settle in for a 20-minute soak. You can buy both herbs in health food stores.

## WOMAN TO WOMAN
### She Found the Snore Cure

*For nearly four decades, Julie Switzer, a postal clerk in Hythe, England, never heard the clock ticking in her bedroom. She was unaware of the garbage truck rumbling down the street, the yowl of prowling cats, and other noises of the night. She was deaf to everything but her husband Melvyn's snoring—which, at 92 decibels, was about as loud as heavy traffic or a thunderstorm in her room. But thanks to a homeopathic remedy, Melvyn and Julie now sleep peacefully side by side.*

Melvyn and I had been married about 10 years when he developed complications from dental surgery and began to snore. I'm deaf in one ear. But even if I took out my hearing aid, put in earplugs, and slept with my good ear down on the pillow, the snoring still got through.

One day I saw an ad in the local paper for a competition to find the loudest snorer. When I asked Mel if he'd mind if I entered him in the contest, he said, "Why? I don't snore." But I entered him anyway.

Of the five snorers picked for the finals, Mel snored loudest at 52 decibels. The intrigued reporter set up another measurement where Mel reached 82.5 decibels. Next came David Frost's Guinness records TV program, where Mel snored at a sonorous 87.5 decibels. Finally, he made *The Guinness Book of Records* at an earsplitting 92 decibels. At that point, Mel acknowledged that he did, in fact, snore.

"Remedies" arrived, unsolicited. People sent all sorts of gadgets—everything from a World War II–type gas mask to a wristband that gave Mel an electric shock when he snored. That one hit the garbage dump quickly.

Then Mel tried all-natural homeopathic antisnoring drops containing just two active ingredients—*Dioscorea villosa* (wild yam) and *Zingiber officinale* (common ginger). Lying on the sofa for a nap, he was *so* quiet. When I told him, he insisted it was a fluke. But that night, he used the drops again. Dead silence. It was spooky for me. Miraculously, it worked the first time and every time since then.

What surprises me is how different *I* feel. I didn't realize how tired and lackadaisical I was until I began to wake up refreshed. Now we both feel much more fit.

# Fight Fatigue

Tired. Pooped. Drained. Weary. Exhausted. Those are just some of the adjectives women use to describe how they feel during a good part of their days. Some say they're tired when they get up in the morning. Others run out of steam in the middle of the afternoon. Still others feel so exhausted all day, every day, that they feel totally out of control of their lives.

For many women, the cause is obvious: They have much to do and too little time to do it. "So many things demand our attention and pull us in different directions that our brains and bodies can't keep pace," says Susan Schenkel, Ph.D., a clinical psychologist in Cambridge, Massachusetts, and author of *Giving Away Success: Why Women Get Stuck and What to Do about It.*

Dr. Schenkel blames this kind of fatigue on what she calls stimulus overload. Unfortunately, a lot of women don't even recognize that they're overburdened. "They just accept what they're doing as normal," she explains. "It doesn't occur to them to take a step back and say, 'Wait a minute, I'm doing way too much.'"

Of course, plenty of other things can wipe you out. A poor night's sleep or a heavy meal can leave you dragging temporarily. More persistent, profound fatigue can be linked to stress, poor nutrition, lack of exercise, or even certain medications. It can also signal an illness such as iron-deficiency anemia or problems with the thyroid gland.

Left to its own devices, fatigue can rob you of your lust for life. Don't let that happen. You can fight it and win.

If none of the following methods help and you've felt overwhelming fatigue for more than a month for no obvious reason, see your doctor. She can determine whether you have an underlying health problem that calls for medical treatment.

## All-Purpose Energy Boosters

The amount of energy you have or don't have has a great deal to do with how you nourish your body and brain. The following habits, practiced daily, should keep you going and going all day long.

**Get an extra 20 minutes of sleep a day.** Either go to bed earlier, sleep later, or take a nap in the afternoon. Studies show that on any given day, half the men and women in the country are walking around sleep-deprived. If you're one of them, then you're probably not functioning on all pistons.

On average, women need between 8 and 8½ hours of sleep a night. (Incidentally, that's 1 to 1½ hours more than men.)

**Delegate at least one chore to someone else.** And don't feel guilty about it. "Compared with men, women tend to place a lot more pressure on themselves," says Dr. Schenkel. "And if we finally do realize that we have to give up something, we feel guilty about it. We worry that our husbands or kids or bosses or cats will feel that they're getting shortchanged." So pick a chore and give it to someone else. Your body and brain will thank you.

**Move your butt—and your arms and legs.** It's a vicious cycle: The more exhausted you feel, the less you feel like getting out and walking the dog, gardening, or taking a stroll. But in an ironic twist of nature, the more you exercise, the less tired you'll feel and the more energy you'll have at the end of the day. So set aside 30 minutes a day, at least three days a week, for some kind of exercise, even if it's just walking.

**Skip candy, cookies, baked goods, and other treats.** A diet replete with treats leaves you sluggish in three ways: Treats crowd out the nutritious foods your body needs, so you may be low on vital nutrients. The fat and sugar they supply wreak havoc with your metabolism and can leave you fatigued. And the extra calories pack on pounds, leaving you feeling like you're walking through mud carrying a 25-pound sack of kitty litter.

---

### REAL-LIFE SCENARIO

### *She Won't Find Energy in This Pill*

Ever since she was a teenager, Audrey has been blessed with supercharged energy. Up early and to bed late, Audrey was on the go all day and out most nights. Balancing work, family, household, and an active social life was no problem for her. Now that she's pushing 40, Audrey is starting to feel herself fade. Most nights now, she'd rather snooze on the sofa than go out to a meeting. And she doesn't like it. Audrey heard about a supplement called spirulina that's supposed to be a natural energy booster, and she has started to take it. She has also doubled up on her vitamins. She wonders, "How soon can I expect to see results?"

Audrey is wasting her money if she thinks that she can find her lost energy simply by taking a supplement. While spirulina, a form of blue-green algae, is touted to boost mental energy, there is no medical proof that it works. And unless she's actually deficient in vitamins and minerals, she's not going to feel a boost by doubling her daily multivitamin. In fact, doubling up on her vitamins could put her health in jeopardy. Many vitamins and minerals, such as vitamins A and D, can be toxic when taken in large doses.

Truth is, what Audrey is experiencing is quite natural. At the age of 40, she shouldn't expect to be revving at the speed that she did at age 20. Her superwoman lifestyle is simply catching up with her. She now needs more sleep and a lighter workload, perhaps both on the job and at home, to relieve her stress and fatigue.

*Expert consulted*
*Jennifer Brett, N.D.*
*Naturopathic physician*
*Stratford, Connecticut*

---

**Take a multi every day.** Women don't always eat as well as they should. So stop by your local drugstore, supermarket, or health food store and pick up a multivitamin/mineral tablet that supplies 400 milligrams of magnesium and 25 milligrams of each B vitamin (including folic acid), nutrients needed to maintain energy.

*Caution:* People with heart or kidney problems should check with their doctors before taking supplemental magnesium. Supplemental magnesium may cause diarrhea in some people.

Your body needs magnesium to get energy from food. And deficiencies of B vitamins, especially $B_{12}$, have been linked to fatigue and memory loss, among other symptoms. Taking supplements with food will help you absorb them better.

**Choose ginseng.** Ginseng has long had a reputation as an energy enhancer, and new research seems to bear this out. The herb is sold in many different forms and potencies. Find a supplement that contains 100 to 125 milligrams of ginseng extract, standardized to contain 4 to 7 percent ginsenosides. (Ginsenosides are said to be the active ingredient in ginseng.)

*Note:* Don't take ginseng without your doctor's okay if you have high blood pressure.

**Become fluent in fluids.** You might not think of water as a nutrient. But water constitutes about 60 percent of your body weight. Your body depends on fluid to function well. Dehydration can sap your energy and impair mental and physical performance. To ensure that you're well-hydrated, fill an empty two-liter bottle with water every morning and take frequent sips throughout the day.

## Afternoon Slump

You don't even have to look at the clock: You know precisely when it's 3:00 P.M. Your eyelids get droopy, your head starts to nod, and your entire body is begging to lie down for just a few minutes.

The urge to snooze in the midafternoon is definitely irresistible—and altogether natural. As

**WOMEN ASK WHY**

*Why is it so hard to get out of bed in the morning, even if I get enough sleep?*

Assuming that you're sleeping a solid eight hours a night, your inability to drag yourself out of bed could have several causes. A woman's normal hormonal fluctuations can interfere with sleep. Women with premenstrual syndrome (PMS) often find it difficult to fall or stay asleep during the week before their periods. The first trimester of pregnancy raises a woman's levels of progesterone, which can cause excessive sleepiness and fatigue in some women. During menopause, declining estrogen levels trigger hot flashes and night sweats. Both can wake a woman out of a sound sleep.

You could have sleep apnea, a condition in which you stop breathing in your sleep for at least 10 seconds at a time. This is more common in men than in women, however. Two other sleep disorders that are more common to women are restless leg syndrome, which is characterized by a restless or jumpy feeling in the legs that makes getting to sleep difficult, and periodic limb movement disorder (PLMD), characterized by a periodic jerking of the legs during sleep. PLMD can wake you dozens of times a

sleep researchers explain it, the human body is programmed for one long sleep period and one short sleep period every 24 hours. The short period occurs 12 hours after the halfway point of the longer period. So if you go to bed at 11:00 P.M. and wake up at 7:00 A.M., you'll likely feel sleepy around 4:00 in the afternoon.

To counteract a midday energy slump, women doctors recommend these quick pick-me-ups.

**Stretch your legs.** Nothing recharges your batteries better than exercise. So when you feel sluggishness setting in, lace up your sneakers and head out for a brisk walk around the block. Just 20 minutes of walking can energize you for up to eight hours afterward.

night, keeping you in a light and not-very-restful stage of sleep.

If you're tired when you get up in the morning, the first thing you should do is examine your sleeping habits and get back on schedule. Your body clock, the part of your brain that regulates sleep needs and patterns, craves regularity. It gets confused when you get out of bed at 7:00 A.M. one morning and at 10:00 A.M. the next.

Exercise helps, too. It makes you sleep more soundly because it tires your body and reduces anxiety that may interfere with sleep.

If you still can't get out of bed, consider consulting a sleep disorders clinic. (They're covered by most insurance.) During your first visit, specialists will take a "sleep history." You may be asked to spend a night or two at the clinic so your sleep can be monitored. In any case, the specialists can make recommendations that can, in time, make getting out of bed a joy rather than a chore.

*Expert consulted*
*Lauren Broch, Ph.D.*
*Director of education and training*
*New York Hospital–Cornell Medical Center*
*Sleep-Wake Disorders Center*
*New York City*

a few seconds, then breathe out, releasing the air slowly and deliberately.

**Sample an energizing aroma.** Put a drop or two of peppermint or rosemary essential oil on a handkerchief. Then sniff the scent for an on-the-spot lift. You can buy essential oils in health food stores and bath-and-beauty shops.

**Focus on your feet.** Use your knuckles to press on the center of the arch of one foot for a few seconds. Repeat on your other foot. According to practitioners of reflexology (the practice of stimulating different parts of the body via selected pressure points, usually on the hands and feet), stimulating this area of the foot wakes you up.

**Capitalize on break time.** For your P.M. coffee break, pair your cup of java with a high-carbohydrate food such as three gingersnaps or four small fig bars. Caffeine provides a mental boost, while carbohydrates trigger the production of serotonin, a brain chemical that keeps you relaxed and focused.

**Roll those shoulders.** Shoulder rolls relieve tension and provide a quick energy boost. To begin, inhale and squeeze your shoulders forward, as though you were collapsing your chest. Next, shrug your shoulders toward your ears. Then exhale and push your shoulders backward, moving your shoulder blades toward each other. Finally, drop your shoulders and relax.

**Take a few deep breaths.** Shallow breathing delivers less air to your lungs per breath, triggering changes that deliver less oxygen to your brain, heart, and the rest of your body. The result is grogginess.

To recharge your energy stores, breathe in through your nose as deeply as you can. Hold for

## Concentration Problems

You know the feeling: You have to get something done, but your brain has other ideas. It keeps wandering off to the shopping list you need to get done or to the glorious weather just outside your window.

Poor concentration could mean that you're bored with what you're doing. But it could also mean that you're too tired to pay attention. Here's how you can keep your thoughts on track.

**Breathe in, breathe out.** Besides boosting oxygen levels, deep breathing also dispels feelings of anxiety that can disrupt your concentration.

**Get in tune with Bach.** For some, listening to baroque music seems to boost concentration.

## FOLK REMEDY: DOES IT WORK?

### Counting Sheep to Fall Asleep

It's the classic sleep-inducing vision: Little white sheep, one by one, jumping over a fence. No one seems to know who dreamed it up, but it makes a lot of sense.

Counting anything can help clear your mind of nagging thoughts and send you off to dreamland, says Susan Zafarlotfi, Ph.D., clinical director of the Institute of Sleep/Wake Disorders at Hackensack University Medical Center in New Jersey.

Counting and visualizing something pleasant—be it sheep, butterflies, or anything else—is a form of guided imagery, a practice that's known to help release stress and anxiety, notes Dr. Zafarlotfi. (So, maybe it was some psychologist who started the sheep-counting.) And being stress-free and clearheaded before bed is a requirement for restful sleep.

Counting sheep may be especially useful for women who often have trouble falling asleep because they're preoccupied with everyday worries and pressures, says Dr. Zafarlotfi.

**RECOMMENDATION:** Worth a Try

Research has shown that the works of German composer Johann Sebastian Bach are especially conducive to learning.

**Eat often.** Consuming frequent small meals keeps your blood sugar levels steady. And that keeps you clearheaded and sharp.

**Select a smart snack.** When your concentration begins to flag, eat a snack that pairs protein with carbohydrates—tuna on whole-wheat bread, for example. The protein/carb combination helps sustain alertness.

**Take a break.** Sometimes poor concentration is your brain's way of telling you that you need a change of pace or a change of scenery or both. A quick walk around the block may be enough to shake off the cobwebs.

**Think ginkgo.** Research has shown that ginkgo biloba extract (GBE) improves concentration in people with cognitive deficiency, a condition caused by inadequate blood flow to and nerve damage in the brain. Look for a GBE product that's labeled "24/6." This tells you that the product contains 24 percent flavone glycosides and 6 percent terpenes. Take 120 to 240 milligrams of GBE in two or three separate doses every day. Keep in mind that the herb works slowly. Give it at least eight weeks to do its stuff.

## Insomnia

Do you have trouble falling asleep at night? Do you fall asleep just fine, but wake up during the night and then find yourself unable to get back to sleep? Do you wake up wide-awake hours before you need to?

If any of these scenarios describes you, then welcome to the club. You, along with roughly one-third of all the other women in America, have insomnia. Women seem to be especially prone, primarily due to hormonal changes that occur during menstruation, pregnancy, and menopause.

Here's how to relax your mind and body for sweet slumber when you want it.

**Get tea'd off.** A number of herbs have properties that calm the nerves and foster sound sleep. Among the herbs to try are kava kava, St.-John's-wort, and valerian. To make a tea, add one tablespoon of dried herb to one cup of freshly boiled water. Allow the tea to steep for an hour, then strain and reheat before drinking. Drink a cup in the morning, one at noon, and one at night so that you're relaxed by the time you go to bed. Don't take valerian during the day, however, because it has a sedative effect. You can buy any of these herbs in health food stores.

**Replace animal protein with soy protein.** Soy foods are rich in phytoestrogens, which can relieve premenopausal symptoms like heat-induced insomnia. You can substitute soy milk in all your cooking, soy cheese for dairy cheese, and tofu for ground meat.

**Snooze in the afternoon.** If your erratic sleeping pattern has really thrown you off-schedule and you feel like you must nap, limit yourself to a half-hour snooze in the middle of the afternoon. Sleep for more than a half-hour, and your body will likely go into a deep-sleep phase that will leave you feeling groggy when you awaken.

**Draw a bath.** Soaking in a comfortably hot bath early in the evening causes your body temperature to rise. Then when you go to bed, your temperature quickly drops. This helps you fall asleep more easily.

**Skip late-night noshing.** Avoid eating a big meal less than four hours before bedtime. Otherwise, digestion—or indigestion—will keep you awake.

**Exercise early.** Working out may tire you out, but not in a way that's conducive to sleeping. Your body needs adequate time to recuperate from the exertion. Schedule your workout for at least three hours before bedtime.

**Relax before retiring.** Before going to bed, allow yourself at least 45 minutes of quiet time. Do some light reading (no suspense novels allowed), listen to soft music, or talk to your cat.

**Create the right environment.** Many people sleep best in a room that's on the cool side. So turn down the thermostat a few degrees before crawling between the sheets. Also, keep your bedroom dark and quiet.

## Iron-Deficiency Anemia

Researchers have identified some 90 different types of anemia. But among women of reproductive age, iron-deficiency anemia is the most common. The primary cause is menstruation. Menstruation depletes your body's supply of iron. When you run low on iron, your body produces fewer and smaller red blood cells. There is less hemoglobin, which means there is less oxygen floating around your bloodstream. This lack of oxygen leaves you feeling exhausted.

Mothers-to-be are prime candidates for anemia, as blood is diverted to the developing fetus and then lost during childbirth.

Some women become iron-deficient not because of menstruation but because of poor eating habits. They're not consuming enough lean meats, soy products, legumes, and other iron-rich foods. Women who crash-diet are especially at risk.

While fatigue is a common symptom of iron-deficiency anemia, it's not the only one. You may also experience shortness of breath, dizziness, lightheadedness, and poor resistance to infection. If you're tired and don't know why, see your doctor for proper diagnosis.

Anemia doesn't go away overnight. With treatment, you may feel better in a few weeks, but you'll need months to adequately replenish your iron stores. Visit your doctor again if you don't feel better after a month of treatment.

The following measures, in addition to any treatment your doctor recommends, can help you overcome anemia.

**Feature meat at one meal.** Meat is the richest source of iron and the primary source of heme iron, which is easily absorbed compared to the nonheme form found in plant-derived foods. Choose lean cuts such as flank steak, sirloin, and top round. Or buy cheaper cuts, such as strip steak and chuck steak, and trim the fat. Aim to eat one three-ounce serving of beef a day.

**Experience the joy of soy.** If you eat little or no meat, you'll need to depend on plant-derived foods for your iron. In general, soy foods and legumes are your best bet because they provide adequate protein levels to ensure that your iron count remains high enough. Another top-notch source is Cream of Wheat cereal. You may also get a kick out of quinoa, a plant protein similar to rice, which is available in health food stores.

**Get juiced.** Studies have found that vitamin C helps boost the absorption of nonheme iron found in plant-based foods. So when you're eating these types of foods, chase them with a glass of orange juice whenever possible.

**Stock your iron stores.** Most experts advise that you check with your doctor before taking iron supplements, to make sure that you actually need them. (Too much iron isn't always healthy either). If you do need iron, take 300 milligrams of ferrous sulfate every day for seven days only during menstruation. These supplements deliver the iron you need when you need it most, but without the risk of toxic buildup. They're available in drugstores without a prescription. Avoid taking them with milk or with food of any kind, which can actually inhibit iron absorption.

**Shed the coating.** If your doctor recommends iron supplements, look for a brand that is not enteric-coated. Your body can better absorb the iron from uncoated tablets.

## Jet Lag

Flying across time zones may be exciting for the psyche, but it's exhausting on the body. That's because as your body greets a new day in a

## WOMAN TO WOMAN
### *Exercise Cured This Couch Potato*

*Charlotte Purvis, 47, a communications coach and motivational speaker in Durham, North Carolina, broke her cycle of fatigue by making a mind/body connection. Here's her story.*

To say that I used to hate to exercise is an understatement. In high school, I negotiated my way out of gym class by agreeing to take geometry. I got straight A's in the class all year because I was afraid the administration would put me back in the gym if I didn't.

As I grew older, I avoided at all cost anything remotely close to exercise. My friends and family knew that whenever they drove me anywhere, I had to be dropped off at the front door. I didn't like walking through a parking lot. My lack of exercise and bad eating habits (I existed mostly on processed foods and sweets) left me constantly tired and with frequent headaches. I gained so much weight that I felt like I was dragging myself through each day, even though I needed at least 10 hours of sleep every night.

Then the day came when I was faced with my upcoming 20-year high school reunion. I became emotional just thinking about seeing everyone from my high school, and I thought long and hard about the young woman I had been.

new place and new time, its internal clock remains set on the old time.

Generally, to reset its clock, your body requires one full day for every time zone crossed. In the meantime, you may experience an array of jet lag symptoms—not just sleep disturbances and fatigue but also headaches, digestive upset, and irritability. Interestingly, traveling from west to east seems to cause more problems than traveling from east to west because you're pushing your body's clock forward instead of back.

But you can't wait three days to unwind when you're on a long weekend to the coast. Besides, vacation time is too precious to waste. Here's

I realized that my years of avoiding exercise had created a huge gap between the way I wanted to feel and the way I actually felt, being almost 40 and seriously out of shape. I knew I needed to make a change.

My husband suggested mall walking. I could barely make it around the one-third-mile stretch of mall. But instead of giving up, I continued. After a couple of weeks, my body started getting stronger, responding to the new movements.

Gradually, I also began to exercise with various yoga and low-impact aerobic programs on television. I felt comfortable working out at my own pace in the privacy of my home. And as my strength and stamina improved, my energy levels skyrocketed. I also began to feel more alert and engaged in my everyday activities. By the time I got to the reunion, I felt comfortable in my body—and my husband says I looked a lot like I did when we first met.

Learning how to exercise has been a long, hard process. I still consider myself to be in the process of getting in shape, and the range of activities I enjoy continues to expand. I've just added biking and toning exercises to my list of favorites. When I think about how good I feel, how much better my energy level is, I think about how happy people look on television when they learn they've just won the jackpot. I feel like a million bucks.

what to do to make jet lag a minor blip in your travel schedule.

**Step outside.** If you arrive at your destination during daylight, head outdoors for some light activity as soon as you can to give your body a chance to acquaint itself with the new time zone. The activity will help your circadian rhythms, your body's natural time-keeping cycle, adjust to your new schedule. A walk around the block is sufficient.

**Spend time in the sun.** Because the day/night cycle governs your body's clock, getting some sun exposure can expedite the adjustment. But you have to time it right. A good rule of thumb: If you fly from west to east, head outside at the morning and retreat indoors by late afternoon. If you fly from east to west, stay indoors in the morning and go outside in the late afternoon.

**Follow the locals' lead.** The first day in your destination, eat and sleep according to the new time. Have dinner at 5:00 P.M. and go to bed at 11:00 P.M., even if it's much earlier or later than your home time.

**Be gentle to your digestion.** Give your digestive system a chance to adjust to the new time zone, too. At least at first, stick with light meals consisting of familiar foods. After a day or two, your stomach will be prepared should you decide to sample some more exotic fare.

**Enjoy a java jolt.** Caffeine can ease your body through the time zone transition, as long as you use it prudently. If you're flying from the West Coast to the East Coast, for example, have a cup of coffee with breakfast on the first morning in your destination. The caffeine can help compensate for the fact that you've essentially lost six hours of sleep. But don't rely on cup after cup of coffee to power you through the day, or you may find yourself the victim of caffeine overload.

**Catch a catnap.** If your body craves a nap, take one. Just make sure that your snooze lasts no longer than a half-hour. Sorry, but no napping after 5:00 P.M. It could prevent you from getting a good night's sleep.

**Skip the cocktails.** While alcohol may seem like the perfect antidote for preflight jitters, it can actually cause more trouble than it's worth. Alcohol affects your central nervous system and can interfere with sleep patterns. Wait a day to enjoy your bon voyage toast.

# Conquer Colds and Infections

**G**erms. They're everywhere—on the phone, on the doorknob, and on the toilet handle. They travel home from the day care center, sail by you from a sneeze in aisle 11 at the supermarket, and shake your hand in the receiving line. They're in the air anyplace, anywhere.

We can't avoid germs, but we certainly can resist them. Truth is, it's the strength of our immune systems that determines who among us will and will not come down with the season's colds and flu. And as women, we leave ourselves open as easy targets.

Women are particularly prone to infections because we're inclined to put the needs of others above our own, says Susanna Cunningham-Rundles, Ph.D., associate professor of immunology at the New York Hospital–Cornell Medical Center in New York City.

"There seems to be an attitude that if you're responsible for others, then you're somehow stronger than everyone else and you don't have to worry about your health," says Dr. Cunningham-Rundles. Actually, as doers of all things for all people, women need to take care of their own health even more.

The first place to start building your immunity is right in the kitchen. "There's no substitute for eating right, and that means plenty of nutrition-packed foods like fruits and vegetables," says Dr. Cunningham-Rundles. She advocates "adding in"—that is, incorporating something healthful into your diet before taking out something unhealthful. That way, changing your eating habits won't feel like punishment.

Supplement your diet with immune-system-building antioxidants—vitamins C and E and beta-carotene—especially around the time of your period, when your immune system is more vulnerable to infection. Exercise builds immunity, so get out there and move for at least 30 minutes three or four times a week. And if you smoke, quit. Smokers are much more likely to get the flu or a respiratory infection than non-smokers are. Last but not least, practice what you tell your kids to do: Wash your hands frequently throughout the day.

If the bug does get you, make sure to drink plenty of liquids, avoid rich foods (they're hard to digest), and get plenty of rest. Plus, you can speed recovery of specific infections by following these natural remedies.

## Bronchitis

Green phlegm is the clue that says you have bronchitis. *Bronchitis* literally means inflammation of the bronchi, the tubes that connect your windpipe and lungs.

Bronchitis can be either acute or chronic. While both kinds make you feel equally miserable, they progress quite differently. Acute bronchitis usually results from an especially persistent cold or flu virus. It can clear up on its own and shouldn't last more than a week. Chronic bronchitis is usually associated with smoking. It can drag on for months or come and go for years. It's serious enough to require a doctor's care.

With either type of bronchitis, getting all that mucus up and out of your lungs is important because mucus-filled lungs are a potential breeding ground for bacteria that cause pneumonia. The following remedies can help clear your lungs and keep you comfortable while the virus runs its course. If your symptoms persist after two days of self-care, see your doctor.

**Hit the shower.** A comfortably hot shower or bath helps loosen stubborn phlegm. It won't make the virus go away any faster, but it'll sure make you feel better.

**Treat your feet.** Instead of a hot shower, try a hot footbath. Soak your feet for 10 minutes. The heat helps draw congestion away from your head, neck, and lungs.

*Note:* Don't use this remedy if you have diabetes or any condition that affects circulation.

**Make a mug of mullein tea.** The herb mullein, a member of the snapdragon family, can help rid your lungs of mucus. To make a tea, steep about two teaspoons of dried mullein leaves in a pot of freshly boiled water for about 10 minutes. Strain the tea, then allow it to cool slightly before drinking it. Repeat three times a day. You can buy dried mullein leaves in health food stores.

**Increase your vitamin C.** Research shows that vitamin C reduces the severity of viral infections, including bronchitis. Take 2,000 milligrams a day in supplement form at the first sign of illness and continue for a few days after you feel better.

*Note:* Some people develop diarrhea when taking large doses of vitamin C. If this happens to you, cut back your daily dosage to 1,000 milligrams or less until the problem subsides.

**Rest your bones.** That achy, tired-all-over feeling is your body's way of telling you to slow down so that it can heal itself. Listen to it. Stay home from work if necessary.

## Colds

Despite amazing advances in modern medicine, not to mention the more than 800 cold remedies on the market today, scientists have yet to identify a cure for this common malady.

Cold medicines, however, aren't totally useless. They help tame the symptoms. But they do carry a host of side effects, such as drowsiness and dry mouth.

If you want relief without the cost and side effects of over-the-counter drugs, try these natural remedies. (See your doctor if you have a cold with a fever over 101°F for more than a couple days or if your cough worsens.)

**Start with zinc.** Taking zinc gluconate lozenges at the first sign of a cold may reduce the duration of your symptoms. Researchers suspect that zinc may work by thwarting viral replication or preventing a virus from entering cells. You can buy zinc gluconate lozenges in health food stores and drugstores.

**Try echinacea.** In the body, echinacea stimulates disease-fighting white blood cells to fend

## FOLK REMEDY: DOES IT WORK?

### Chicken Soup for a Cold

Even the ancient Egyptians were on to this one. Maimonides, the twelfth century physician and philosopher who spent most of his life in Egypt, recommended chicken soup for a fever and cough.

While no one has claimed that chicken soup can cure a cold, it can make you feel better. "Chicken soup is a form of hydrotherapy for your throat," says Angela Stengler, N.D., a naturopathic physician in Oceanside, California. Inhaling the steam from a hot bowl of soup—or sipping any hot liquid—will increase blood flow to the affected area. White blood cells can then get there quickly and start fighting infection faster. "And it increases and loosens mucus flow from your nose," she adds.

Chicken soup can also boost your energy when you're feeling lousy. "If you're sick and not eating, your blood sugar level will fall, making you feel worse," she says. "Food raises your blood sugar and makes you feel better."

You can fortify your chicken soup with cold-fighting herbs, such as garlic and ginger. "Garlic is antibacterial, antifungal, and antiviral," notes Dr. Stengler, "while ginger calms the stomach and is a decongestant." You can also spice up your soup with hot peppers, which help increase circulation and get those white blood cells moving.

**RECOMMENDATION:** Worth a Try

multiple sclerosis, don't use echinacea at all. Same goes if you're allergic to other plants in the daisy family, like chamomile.

**Reach for garlic.** Garlic has potent antibiotic and antiviral properties, so taking it in supplement form may minimize cold symptoms. Look for enteric-coated garlic capsules in health food stores. The usual dosage is 300 milligrams three times a day until symptoms subside. Or if you like yours raw, eat $1\frac{1}{2}$ cloves each day.

**Drink a lot.** A lot of water, that is. Your body uses up fluids when fighting a cold virus, so staying hydrated is critical. Make sure that you're drinking at least eight eight-ounce glasses of water a day. Steer clear of sweetened fruit juices and sodas, though. They act as diuretics, flushing water out of your system.

**Elevate your head.** Propping your head on pillows when you lie down makes breathing easier, especially if you have postnasal drip.

## Congestion

Forget the fact that it feels like someone put a plastic bag over your head. When you're stuffed up, food tastes like toilet paper. You can't taste a thing.

You can relieve occasional bouts of congestion on your own. If you frequently feel congested or stuffy and you're not getting better, check in with your doctor. Same goes if congestion is accompanied by green or yellow phlegm, severe headache or facial pain, fever, or persistent cough.

Here's what to do to nip this problem in the bud real fast.

off cold viruses. The herb is available in a variety of forms in health food stores and some drugstores. Look for capsules that supply 125 milligrams of echinacea extract, standardized to contain 4 percent total echinacosides (the herb's active ingredients).

*Note:* Don't use echinacea continuously for more than 12 weeks, to give your body a break. If you have an autoimmune disease like lupus or

**Get steamed.** Pour three cups of water into a pot and bring it to a simmer. Remove the pot from the stove and set it where you can sit in front of it, such as on your kitchen table. Lean over the pot and drape a towel over your head. (Don't put your face too close to the steam, though, or you may burn yourself.) Inhale the steam for five minutes. This should help loosen the mucus in clogged nasal passages.

**Mix a scented rub.** Camphor, eucalyptus, and menthol are natural decongestants. You can make a rub from any of these essential oils by mixing a couple drops in a handful of corn oil. Put it on your temples, beneath your nose, on your neck—anywhere you can smell it. Essential oils are sold in health food stores and bath-and-beauty shops. If it irritates your skin, don't use it.

**Heat up your meals.** Hot pepper helps open clogged nasal passages by thinning mucus and making your nose run. Try sprinkling ground red pepper, red-pepper flakes, or hot-pepper sauce on your food.

**Make your own nasal spray.** A homemade saline solution can clear your nose of irritants such as dust, pollen, and pollution. To make the solution, add one-half teaspoon of salt and a pinch of baking soda to one cup of lukewarm water. Spritz the solution into your nose a few times, using a child-size bulb syringe. Then blow your nose.

**Throw the spray away.** Over-the-counter nasal sprays and decongestants may provide

quick relief, but they are really doing you more harm than good. Overuse can cause a rebound effect. In other words, once you stop using them, the stuffiness comes back worse than before. If you use nasal sprays, stop the treatment after three days. Don't use decongestants for more than seven days.

---

### FOLK REMEDY: DOES IT WORK?

**Hot Toddy for Congestion**

The toddy has a long history of being the best cure for congestion, and it seems like just about every old-timer has her version of how to brew one. Basically, it's a hot drink composed of boiling water, a sweetener, and spices, spiked with a shot of liquor.

Even the teetotaling Amish have a congestion remedy using whiskey to which they add lemon, flaxseeds, and hot water, then—for good measure—some brandy. Another classic toddy is hot buttered rum, consisting of brown sugar, cloves, boiling water, a dab of butter, and a jigger of rum, stirred with a cinnamon stick.

Does the toddy work? Yes, if you omit the alcohol, says Susan Calvert Finn, R.D., Ph.D., director of nutrition at Roth Laboratories in Columbus, Ohio, and author of *The American Dietetic Association Guide to Women's Nutrition for Healthy Living*. Although liquor can help bring on the virus-fighting sweats, it stresses your immune system. It can also temporarily increase nasal congestion. And alcohol is initially a stimulant—not exactly the gentle treatment required when your nose is sore, your eyes burn, and you need a long winter's nap.

So mix up a hot toddy without the alcohol to soothe your swollen membranes and help break up mucus. Add a tea bag of chamomile or peppermint leaves to boost the soothing qualities, and be sure to inhale the steam to lubricate your nasal passages.

**RECOMMENDATION:** Worth a Try

## Coughing

Think of it as a necessary evil. Coughing clears your airways of mucus, phlegm, and other undesirable matter that you'd much rather be without.

Of course, this bit of knowledge provides little comfort when you're hacking away during a meeting, a church service, or your kid's piano recital. At times like these, you just want to get it under control. Here's how.

**Have some licorice.** The sweet taste of licorice—the herb, not the candy—soothes the throat. And, according to studies, it suppresses the cough reflex. To make a tea, add one-half teaspoon of licorice root to one cup of freshly boiled water. Allow to steep for 10 minutes, then strain and allow to cool slightly before drinking.

*Note:* Don't take licorice more than three times a day or for more than two weeks, especially if your blood pressure tends to be high.

**Take your thyme.** Thyme is a natural antimicrobial and expectorant. It also relaxes airway muscles, which helps stymie a cough. To make a tea, pour six ounces of freshly boiled water over 1 2/3 teaspoons of fresh thyme leaves or 1/2 or 2/3 teaspoon of dried leaves. (Use medicinal-quality thyme from a health food store, not the thyme in your spice rack.) Cover and steep for 10 minutes, then strain and allow to cool slightly before drinking. Repeat three times a day for up to three days.

**Drink carrot juice.** Put a few drops of vegetable oil in a glass of fresh carrot juice, then take frequent sips throughout the day. Carrots are loaded with vitamin A, which strengthens your respiratory system and can quiet your cough. The vegetable oil coats and soothes your throat.

## Ear Infections

Kids may corner the market when it comes to ear infections, but that doesn't mean that grown-ups can't get them, too.

Many doctors recommend antibiotics for any type of ear infection for two reasons. First, a severe infection, left untreated, can lead to hearing loss. Second, a severe infection could spread to structures close to the ear, causing more serious problems.

So if you suspect that you have an ear infection, see your doctor. Then use these home remedies in conjunction with antibiotic treatment to quickly relieve ear pain and discomfort.

**Feel the heat.** Hold a hot-water bottle, a hot towel, or a heating pad over the affected ear for up to 20 minutes. (If you're using a hot-water bottle or a heating pad, warm it to a comfortably hot temperature and wrap it in a towel before applying it.) Heat stimulates blood flow, which alleviates pain. It also marshals white blood cells, your body's infection-fighters, to the ear area.

**Add a little mullein oil.** An oil extract made from the herb mullein, a member of the snapdragon family, has potent antibacterial properties. Put a bottle of the oil (sold in most health food stores) in a small pan of water and carefully heat it over low heat until it's warm but not hot. Gently shake the bottle, then put a drop or two of the oil on your wrist. If the temperature feels comfortable, use an eyedropper to put a drop of the oil in the affected ear. To coax the drops into your ear, gently pull your ear back and up to straighten the ear canal. Plug the ear's opening with a wad of cotton. Repeat two or three times a day until the infection clears. Don't use this remedy if your eardrum is perforated.

**Take a deep breath.** The deep-breathing techniques practiced in Qigong, a Chinese healing discipline, may help relieve ear pain. Here's one to try: Imagine that the area from behind your naval to your upper chest is an accordion. Inhale through your nose to fill this area with air and expand the accordion. Then exhale, allowing the air to escape through your lips and collapse the accordion. Continue breathing this way until you feel relaxed and your ear pain subsides. Repeat as needed over a 24-hour period.

**Make your own eardrops.** A homemade concoction of alcohol and vinegar can help clear up swimmer's ear and keep it from coming back. The alcohol evaporates the water trapped inside your ear, while the vinegar kills the infection-causing bacteria. Combine equal parts rubbing alcohol and distilled white vinegar in a clean eyedropper bottle. Use the eyedropper to put a few drops of the solution in the affected ear. To coax the drops into your ear, gently pull your ear back and up to straighten the ear canal. One application may be all you need to cure swimmer's ear, but it's a good idea to use drops after every swim to prevent future infections. (If you've ever punctured your eardrum, this remedy isn't for you.)

## Genital Herpes

Here's something to think about next time you're propositioned by an old flame at your class reunion. One out of every five people has genital herpes.

Some people don't even know they have it because they haven't experienced any of the symptoms, which include a burning sensation and red, pimple-like blisters with watery yellow centers in the genital area. (If you have these signs, see your doctor as soon as possible.) As many as three-quarters of the people who are infected never will have these symptoms.

> ## THE RIGHT WAY TO DE-WAX
>
> Earwax, a goopy composite of glandular secretions, oil, sweat, and dead skin cells, actually serves an important purpose. It traps dirt, dust, and other foreign particles before they travel inside your ear, where they can damage your eardrum, says Jennifer Derebery, M.D., assistant clinical professor of otolaryngology at the University of Southern California and associate of the House Ear Clinic and Institute, both in Los Angeles. But some ears produce too much wax or unusually hard wax. If it isn't removed, it can cause more harm than good, including pain and even temporary hearing loss.
>
> If you have a problem with earwax, Dr. Derebery suggests using baby oil to clear it out. Here's what to do. (If you have a punctured or perforated eardrum, skip this procedure and see your doctor instead.)
>
> 1. Using an eyedropper, place a few drops of room-temperature baby oil in your ear. Repeat twice a day for two or three days. The oil will soften and liquefy the wax.
>
> 2. If the wax doesn't come out on its own, then on the third or fourth day, fill a small bulb syringe with warm water. Pull your ear up and back in the direction of the crown of your head to open up the ear canal. Tilt your head to the side and gently squirt the water into your ear. (If you have especially stubborn wax, you may have to repeat this step a few times.)
>
> 3. Once the wax flows out, put an eyedropper full of a solution of half vinegar and half rubbing alcohol into your ear and let it drain out. This will dry the ear canal and help prevent infection.
>
> Under no circumstances should you use cotton swabs, hairpins, paper clips, or other pointy objects to poke and prod inside your ear, Dr. Derebery cautions. All that does is jam the wax deeper into the ear canal.

Herpes flare-ups should be treated with the prescription antiviral drug acyclovir (Zovirax). With drug therapy, flare-ups may become less frequent and severe and may even stop altogether. While you're waiting for the medicine to work, here's what you can do to ease the discomfort.

**Take an oatmeal bath.** Added to bathwater, colloidal oatmeal quickly soothes the itching and irritation that often accompany a genital herpes flare-up. Look for a colloidal oatmeal bath treatment in your drugstore.

**Don droopy drawers.** Tight-fitting garments, including underpants and panty hose, can cause your skin to chafe. And chafing irritates already-sensitive herpes sores, making them hurt even more. Stick with loose-fitting attire until your sores heal.

**Save sex for later.** Engaging in sexual intercourse during a genital herpes flare-up is a bad idea for several reasons. First, it is quite painful. Second, it puts your partner at risk for infection. And third, it puts you at increased risk for other sexually transmitted diseases, including HIV. Wait until your sores heal before resuming sexual activity, and remember to use latex condoms to protect yourself and avoid infecting your partner.

## WOMAN TO WOMAN

### *She Saved Herself from Sinus Surgery*

*For 15 long years, Rosemary Forrest, 48, of Augusta, Georgia, battled recurrent sinus infections that stemmed from allergies. She constantly felt tired, sluggish, and mentally drained. After years of depending on antibiotics that caused severe stomach upset, Rosemary's doctor suggested that she undergo surgery. Just the word "surgery" sent Rosemary on one of the most important missions of her life. She went on a natural therapy program to heighten her immunity so that she could avoid surgery and stop taking the antibiotics that made her feel so sick all the time. Here is Rosemary's story on how she got her allergies under control—without surgery.*

When the doctor suggested that I get a CAT scan of my sinuses as a preliminary step to surgery, I realized I needed to find another way to feel better. On top of the anxiety over the possibility of surgery, the side effects from the medication I was taking were so severe that I often thought that I would be better off just living with sinus infections. So I started investigating natural alternatives and eventually put together a regimen that I really believe allowed me to achieve the good health I enjoy today.

It started when my daughter had problems with her bladder. Her doctor recommended that she take zinc to improve her immune system. So I began looking into the bene-

## Laryngitis

No one's ever gone mute from laryngitis. The voice usually returns to normal within a few days. But if you have a few things more that you have to say and you just can't wait, try these remedies.

**Reach into the candy jar.** Sucking on a piece of hard candy can be quite soothing. It increases the production of saliva, which wets your parched voice box.

**Make lemon-aid.** Squeeze the juice from one or two fresh lemons. Add a tablespoon of honey and a pinch of ground red pepper. Take a

sip of this concoction every few hours throughout the day. (If your mouth or stomach is very sensitive, skip this remedy.)

**Create a mini-sauna.** Bring three cups of water to a simmer, then remove the pot from the stove. Add one-quarter teaspoon of eucalyptus or peppermint essential oil. Sit or stand so that your face is over the pot. (Don't get too close, though, or you could burn yourself.) Drape a towel over your head and breathe in the steam. Come up for air after five minutes.

**Rely on water.** When you have laryngitis, what feels like phlegm is actually swollen tissues. So frequent ahem-ing to clear your throat only fits of zinc, plus other vitamins and minerals. I started taking zinc, vitamin E, and vitamin C. On alternating days, I would take vitamin A and vitamin D on one day, then beta-carotene on the next day. And if I started to feel sick again, I swallowed an extra capsule of zinc and of vitamin C as a booster. (*Editor's note:* Don't try to follow a regimen like this without consulting your doctor. Taking large amounts of zinc or vitamin E may lead to serious side effects.)

In addition to the vitamins, I took the advice of a friend and purchased a mixture of three essential oils: tea tree, eucalyptus, and peppermint. She said inhaling the oils could keep my nasal passages clear of mucus and, therefore, infection. In the morning when I made myself a cup of tea, I would pour an extra cup of water and spill in a few drops of the oils. As the tea steeped, I would inhale deeply over the cup containing the essential oils. I was amazed by how it helped my ability to breathe. On days when my allergies were particularly bad, I used an over-the-counter saline nasal spray and antihistamines.

I followed this regimen faithfully for about six months. When the next allergy season rolled around, something strange happened: I did not get sick. I was so happy. I felt as if a giant burden had been lifted from on top of me. I finally had my life back.

makes matters worse. Instead, take frequent sips of water for relief.

**Act speechless.** Refrain from speaking while you have laryngitis. If you must speak, keep your voice soft and low-pitched, but don't whisper. Whispering actually strains your vocal cords. Likewise, avoid gargling, because it irritates your vocal cords.

## Sinus Infections

With each of the 23,000 breaths you take per day, you expose your nose to disease-causing viruses and airborne particles of dust, pollen, and smoke. Sometimes these foreign invaders irritate the mucous membrane that lines your nasal passages. The resulting pain and stuffiness are classic symptoms of a sinus infection, also called sinusitis.

Acute sinusitis usually results from a cold or flu virus. While acute sinusitis makes you feel rotten, it's relatively short-lived. It should clear up in 10 to 14 days. Chronic sinusitis, on the other hand, is milder but more persistent and is usually associated with environmental triggers. Symptoms can linger for months.

No matter which type of sinusitis you may have, you can relieve your symptoms with the following self-care measures. If you don't notice any improvement within two weeks, see your doctor.

**Give your nose a workout.** Using your index fingers, press into the small depression on the outside of each nostril. Hold for five seconds, slowly exhaling through your mouth. Then release for five seconds, slowly inhaling through your nose. Repeat several times. This exercise should clear congestion and have you breathing better in minutes.

**Be a hothead.** Applying moist heat improves circulation and delivers vital oxygen and nutrients to your sinuses so that they can heal more quickly. Drape a comfortably hot, moist towel directly over your face, covering the area from the middle of your forehead to your upper lip. Leave the towel in place for 5 to 15 minutes. Repeat twice a day.

**Raise your legs.** Lie on your back with your legs raised against a wall and your buttocks pressed against the wall's base. Stay in this position for 7 to 15 minutes. At first, the pressure in

## WALKING PNEUMONIA: A MISLEADING NAME

If you're walking around with walking pneumonia, you better get off your feet—fast. In fact, if you don't get treatment right away, you may not have any choice.

Walking pneumonia appears as a cold that only gets worse instead of better. It usually begins as an upper-respiratory-tract infection, often with a sore throat, and progresses to a cough within a few days. Later on, you may develop fatigue, malaise, and a low-grade fever. After a week, when it becomes clear that the problem is lingering, it is time to see your doctor. Even though you may not feel all that bad, your sickness will only get worse if you don't determine the cause of the problem and treat it accordingly, says Deirdre O'Connor, N.D., a naturopathic doctor in Mystic, Connecticut.

Even though natural remedies can't cure the problem, they can help you get through it and help keep you from getting it again by keeping your immune system in top shape. Here is what Dr. O'Connor suggests you do.

➤ Take between 1,000 and 3,000 milligrams of vitamin C a day. Eat plenty of high C foods such as broccoli, brussels sprouts, sweet red peppers, sweet potatoes, and citrus fruits. (Some people develop diarrhea with high doses of vitamin C. If this happens to you, reduce your dosage.)

➤ Make sure that your daily multivitamin has 15 milligrams of zinc in it. Immune cells are so dependent on zinc that they can't fight off infection unless they have this mineral. You'll also find zinc in meats, poultry, eggs, dairy products, and oysters.

➤ Brew an immunity soup. Start with a basic vegetable broth, then toss in sweet red peppers, winter squash, carrots, garlic, onions, and any other colorful vegetables. Make this tasty meal frequently during the winter and especially when you are sick. It contains beta-carotene and other carotenoids that enhance the work of the immune system.

➤ Cook with lots of garlic and onions. These two related foods may have antiviral and antibiotic properties, so they can help your immune system fight off both viral and bacterial pneumonia.

your sinuses will increase. But then it will subside as the mucus loosens up. (Avoid this exercise if you have high blood pressure or glaucoma or are at risk for stroke.)

**Drink ginger tea.** Because it's so rich in zinc, ginger can help reduce the inflammation and congestion associated with sinusitis. To make a tea, finely chop a one-quarter-inch slice of fresh ginger and add it to one cup of water in a non-aluminum pot. Cover the pot and let the water boil for 10 to 15 minutes. Strain the tea and allow it to cool slightly before drinking it. Repeat as needed.

*Note:* If you have gallstones, skip this remedy.

**Sip with abandon.** Drinking plenty of water keeps nasal passages moist. Aim for at least eight eight-ounce glasses a day.

**Humidify your environment.** Use a cool-mist humidifier year-round, setting it so that the mist falls close to your face. Be sure to clean the appliance regularly, following the manufacturer's instructions.

## Urinary Tract Infections

One in every five women will contract a urinary tract infection sometime in her life. And once you've had one, you're very likely to get more.

Urinary tract infections produce a few telltale symptoms: a frequent, urgent need to urinate; stinging, burning, or pain when urinating;

passing just a few drops of urine at a time; and passing blood in the urine. Left untreated, these symptoms usually go away on their own in three to seven days.

Women are more susceptible to urinary tract infections right before menstruation and during menopause, most likely because of hormonal changes. Certain birth control methods also appear to increase risk. Diaphragms, for instance, may kink the urethra, preventing the bladder from emptying completely. And spermicides may change the vaginal flora, causing an overgrowth of *Escherichia coli* bacteria.

If you suspect that you have a urinary tract infection, most women doctors recommend that you see your doctor to rule out a more serious problem. She may prescribe antibiotics to kill the bacteria that caused the infection in the first place. In the meantime, these tips can help alleviate your discomfort and prevent future infections.

**Order a baking soda cocktail.** When you feel a urinary tract infection coming on, add one-half teaspoon of baking soda to eight ounces of water and drink the mixture. The baking soda raises the pH (acid-base balance) of irritating, acidic urine.

**Buy berries in a bottle.** An as-yet-unidentified substance in cranberry juice prevents bacteria from adhering to the walls of the urethra and bladder. Drink three eight-ounce glasses of cranberry juice cocktail every day until your infection clears. If you don't like cranberry juice, try blueberry juice instead; it has the same effect.

**Flush out bacteria.** Water increases urine

## WOMEN ASK WHY

### Why are women plagued with more urinary tract infections than men are?

When it comes to urinary tract infections (UTIs), anatomy rules. A woman's urethra, the tube through which urine flows out of one's body, is much shorter than a man's. So any bacteria outside your body can creep up into your bladder much more easily than bacteria can climb the considerably longer male urethra. The bacteria set up shop, and before long, you have a urinary tract infection.

Women also tend to "hold it" longer than men, especially when they are away from home and either don't like the places available to go to the bathroom or have to endure long waits for public restrooms. Putting off urination increases the chances of developing an infection because bacteria aren't getting flushed out as frequently.

After menopause, women have an added strike against them. As women age, the lining of the urethra becomes thinner, allowing bacteria to ascend into the bladder even more easily. So the older you get, the more vigilant you need to be about preventing UTIs.

*Expert consulted*
*Dorothy Barbo, M.D.*
*Medical director of the University Center for*
*    Women's Health*
*University of New Mexico School of Medicine*
*Albuquerque*

flow, washing bacteria out of your urinary tract. As a treatment, drink one eight-ounce glass of water every hour for eight hours.

**Sit in a soothing bath.** To ease the external burning, take a soak in a bath with essential oils and vinegar. In a small dish, combine two tablespoons of honey with the following essential oils, available at health food stores: three drops of sandalwood (an antibacterial), two drops of tea tree (an antiseptic), and one drop of chamomile (an anti-inflammatory). Fill your bathtub halfway with warm or tepid water, then add two tablespoons of apple cider vinegar and the honey–essential oil mixture. Sit and soak for 15 to 20 minutes.

**Raise your C level.** Vitamin C inhibits the growth of bacteria in the urinary tract. Try taking 2,000 milligrams every day for up to three days.

*Note:* Some people develop diarrhea with high doses of vitamin C. If this happens, reduce your dosage until the problem subsides.

## Vaginitis

Vaginitis is known by many names and is caused by many things. But they all produce the same result: burning, itching, discharge, and a whole lot of squirming. The most common form, bacterial vaginosis, occurs when something disturbs the balance among the microorganisms living in the vagina.

Trichomoniasis is the sexually transmitted form of vaginitis. It's caused by a protozoan that gains access to the genitourinary tract. But the best known is the yeast infection, which is caused by an overgrowth of the fungus *Candida albicans* in the vagina.

Vaginitis tends to surface during times of hormonal fluctuation, such as before menstruation and during pregnancy. The risk also rises after menopause, when the vaginal walls become thinner and more vulnerable to infection.

If you experience symptoms of vaginitis, see your doctor. Though vaginitis itself usually isn't serious, it can lead to more serious problems if not properly treated. Your doctor will likely prescribe antibiotics or vaginal cream, which should provide relief in two to three days. The following remedies can help speed relief of itching and discomfort.

**Try the treatment.** Soak a tea bag in water, allow it to cool in the refrigerator, then apply it to the vaginal area. The tannin in the tea can soothe the affected area and relieve itching. (This remedy is intended for external use only.)

**Go for the cold.** Instead of a tea bag, try laying a clean, cold washcloth against the affected area. The cold causes blood vessels to constrict, which reduces inflammation.

**Do a no-soap soak.** Sitting in a shallow sitz bath, or even a regular bath, can soothe the irritated vaginal tissues. But skip the bubbles or any kind of soap, for that matter. It leaches out your skin's natural oils, which protect against germs.

**Eat your yogurt.** If you have bacterial vaginosis, eat eight ounces of yogurt containing live cultures every day to help clear up the infection. The acidophilus bacteria in yogurt helps restore normal bacterial balance in the vagina. Not every yogurt has live cultures, so check the labels.

**Revise your toilet procedure.** When using the toilet, remember to wipe from front to back. This prevents the transfer of germs from the rectal area to the urethra.

**Make a yogurt compress.** For yeast infections, put one-half cup of plain yogurt on a clean cloth or towel. Apply the compress to the vaginal area for 15 minutes. Then rinse off the yogurt with warm water and dry the area with a blow-dryer on the warm setting. The yogurt helps relieve itching. (This remedy is for external use only.)

**Put out the unwelcome mat.** *C. albicans*, often known simply as candida, thrives in a warm, moist environment. To create less hospitable living conditions, wear cotton underwear to stay cool and dry and sprinkle cornstarch in your groin area to absorb moisture.

**Eat carrots.** Eating carrots and other beta-carotene-rich foods may protect against yeast infections by bolstering your immune system.

**Turn sour on sweets.** *C. albicans* loves sugar. When you eat too much of the sweet stuff, the fungus has a feast. So if you're prone to yeast infections, avoid any sugary foods.

# Allergy Relief

**B**iting into a warm slice of wheat toast. The aromatic whiff of a fresh rose. A cuddly little kitten purring next to your knee. Pleasant experiences, for sure, unless you're a woman plagued with allergies.

Allergens are everywhere—from dander on the cat to dust mites on the pillow to certain foods and medicines. No one knows why they rile some people and not others. But genetics seems to play a role. "If one or both of your parents have allergies, then you're much more likely to have allergies, too," says Marianne Frieri, M.D., Ph.D., director of the allergy/immunology training program at Nassau County Medical Center and North Shore University Hospital, both on Long Island.

Hormone changes during pregnancy and menstruation heighten some women's sensitivity to allergens.

If you suspect that you have an allergy, see your doctor. "The trouble is, it takes a qualified doctor and testing to identify what it is you're really allergic to," Dr. Frieri says. Only then can you successfully adjust your lifestyle.

For help with particular allergic conditions, here's what to do.

## Asthma

Asthma is a chronic condition that affects the bronchi (the tubes that carry air in and out of your lungs), making them prone to mucus buildup and infection. Asthma attacks—which include wheezing, coughing, and gasping for air—are usually triggered by something in the environment, such as pet dander, dust mites, molds, pollens, and cigarette smoke, but they can also be brought on by respiratory infections, stress, anger, laughing, crying, and exercise.

During an asthma attack, the inflamed tissues inside your lungs narrow your airways, which become plugged with excess mucus. As the airways swell, the muscles around them constrict, blocking breathing.

Women who have asthma are more prone to attacks before and during their periods, as hormonal fluctuations stimulate mucus production in the nose, throat, and lungs. Asthma also seems to worsen late in the second trimester of pregnancy. But some women have fewer attacks in the month before the baby is due.

If you have asthma, your allergist may prescribe a bronchodilator inhaler. The medicine in the inhaler opens up bronchial passages, allowing you to breathe more easily. In addition, the following self-care measures can help keep you breathing easy.

**In a pinch, quaff coffee.** If you feel an asthma attack coming on and you don't have your inhaler with you, drink a cup or two of coffee instead. Caffeine works fairly well as a bronchodilator.

**Apply pressure.** Make your hands into fists and hold them in front of your chest, thumbs pointing up. Using your thumbs, press along the muscles underneath your collarbone until you feel a knotted, sensitive spot on each side of your chest. Press these points with your thumbs for two minutes, hanging your head forward and breathing slowly and deeply as you do.

**Pressure Points**

**Exhale longer.** Inhale and exhale as you normally do. Then, on the exhalation, continue a bit longer than what feels natural, without forcing out your breath. This yoga breathing technique may serve as a preventive strategy to reduce the number of asthma attacks you experience, according to one study.

**Pay attention to pills.** Certain medications, including aspirin, ibuprofen, and other nonsteroidal anti-inflammatory drugs, can make asthma worse. If you experience more symptoms after starting a new medicine or increasing dosage, tell your doctor.

**Supplement your diet.** Some vitamins and minerals have been found to lessen asthma symptoms. Check with your doctor before adding these to your treatment plan.

&#10003; Magnesium may relax the smooth muscle that lines your airways, minimizing the spasms characteristic of an asthma attack. Nutrition experts recommend 100 to 500 milligrams of magnesium one to three times a day, depending on how much your body can tolerate. Start with the lowest dosage and gradually increase. If you experience symptoms such as gas, cramps, or diarrhea, take less until your symptoms subside.

*Note:* If you have heart or kidney problems, consult your doctor before taking magnesium.

&#10003; Vitamin C may help reduce your coughing and wheezing. Take 1,000 milligrams four times a day. (Excess vitamin C may cause diarrhea in some people.)

&#10003; Quercetin, a bioflavonoid (plant compound), works by inhibiting the mast cells, a component of your immune system that causes allergic reactions by releasing histamine. You can buy quercetin capsules in health food stores. Take 250 milligrams a day.

&#10003; Fish oil can help reduce bronchial inflammation. In addition to adding oily fish like salmon and mackerel to your diet, experts recommend taking 240 milligrams of fish oil in capsule form twice a day.

&#10003; Evening primrose oil may also help reduce inflammation. Capsules are available in health food stores. Take two 500-milligram capsules three times a day. Stop using them if you experience side effects such as headaches, nausea, or diarrhea.

## Eczema

If you have allergies, you may also often have bouts with eczema, a pink, scaly rash that itches intensely. The most common type of eczema is atopic dermatitis, an allergic inflammation of the skin that often affects women who have asthma or hay fever. There's also contact dermatitis, an allergic reaction to an external irritant such as hair coloring or detergent.

While researchers have yet to discover a cure for eczema, doctors suggest these steps for relieving symptoms and minimizing flare-ups.

**Change the way you bathe.** During an eczema flare-up, bathing once or twice a day can make you feel better. But don't soak in hot water. Instead, use lukewarm water and a mild, nonirritating soap. Stay in the tub until your skin starts to pucker and crinkle, a sign that the skin cells have absorbed water and are hydrated.

**Moisturize within three minutes.** To seal in moisture, apply lotion to your skin while it's still damp—within three minutes of your bath or shower. Choose a product with minimal fragrance, color, and additives, all of which can irritate the skin.

**Take some skin-friendly supplements.** Several nutrients can quickly end an eczema flare-up. Take them as needed. All are available in health food stores.

❧ Evening primrose oil contains essential fatty acids, which reduce inflammation. Take two to four

---

### NICKEL ALLERGIES: A DIME A DOZEN

You thought everyone was admiring your beautiful brand-new earrings. But now you realize what they were really staring at were your inflamed, swollen, scaling, oozing earlobes. Where on earth did that nasty rash come from?

You're probably having an allergic reaction to nickel, an ingredient in the metal alloys found in most jewelry as well as in bra hooks, zippers, belt buckles, and metal eyeglass frames. In the United States, about 10 percent of women are allergic to nickel, according to Marianne Frieri, M.D., Ph.D., director of the allergy/immunology training program at Nassau County Medical Center and North Shore University Hospital, both on Long Island.

Curiously, though, many women who react do so only to the nickel in earrings. Experts believe that newly pierced ears may bring out the allergy, but even women who prefer clip-ons can experience problems.

To soothe and heal your irritated earlobes, apply a milk compress, recommends Hilary Baldwin, M.D., associate professor of dermatology and director of dermatologic surgery at the State University of New York Health Science Center at Brooklyn. Pour whole milk into a bowl and add a few ice cubes. Then dip a soft white cloth into the milk, wring it out, and hold it against your ear for 5 to 15 minutes. Do this several times a day. Milk has anti-inflammatory properties, which should help clear up the rash within a matter of days.

Finding earrings that are nickel-free can be a challenge. According to Dr. Baldwin, even those considered "pure" gold contain tiny amounts of nickel. The higher the number of carats, the softer the gold—and the more easily nickel leaches out.

Try wearing earrings made of stainless steel, suggests Dr. Baldwin. They also contain nickel, but the metals are so firmly bound together that the nickel can't leach out.

If you absolutely must wear a pair of allergy-provoking earrings, Dr. Baldwin says that you can reduce your risk of a rash by coating the metal components with clear nail polish. Let the polish dry for 24 hours before putting on the earrings and reapply it each time you wear the earrings.

500-milligram capsules three times a day. Stop using them if you experience side effects such as headaches, nausea, or diarrhea.

❧ Quercetin blocks histamine, the substance released by the skin in response to an allergen. Take two 125-milligram capsules daily.

**Feed on fish.** If you have frequent eczema flare-ups, you may not be getting enough essential fatty acids in your diet. To increase your intake, eat fish rich in omega-3 and omega-6 fatty acids, such as salmon, mackerel, and herring, three or four times a week.

**Give your hands the rubber-glove treatment.** Cleaning products, soap and water, and even dust can trigger a flare-up. So slip on rubber gloves and cotton glove liners when washing dishes and housecleaning.

**Clean clothes carefully.** Use a mild laundry detergent and rinse clothes twice to eliminate detergent residue. And steer clear of scented fabric softeners since the fragrances can irritate your skin.

---

## WOMAN TO WOMAN

### Wheat Is Her Germ

*For years, Pamela Greenfield, a 47-year-old entrepreneur from Great Neck, New York, suffered endless migraines, sore throats, swollen glands, and fatigue. She finally discovered the true cause: a wheat intolerance. Here's how her life without wheat has opened new doors for her.*

Pizza, bagels, pasta. These were the comfort foods I ate whenever I felt lousy, which, for nearly 20 years, was almost every day. But I never realized that by eating these foods, I was practically poisoning myself.

Ever since I was a teenager, I was constantly on some kind of medication for an endless list of problems, including migraine headaches, sore throats, swollen glands, and fatigue. At first I was diagnosed with chronic fatigue syndrome. By the time I was 35, I was so sick that I spent six months in bed and couldn't even walk across the room.

For a while, medication helped. But by the time I was 40, all the old symptoms were back. Someone finally recommended a nutritionist.

The nutritionist started me on a five-day detoxifying regimen. I couldn't eat anything but juice mixed with a rice protein-based nutritional powder containing important nutrients like vitamins A and C, calcium, and iron. I didn't think I could

---

## Food Allergies

When you have a food allergy, your immune system mistakenly identifies certain proteins in foods as a threat to your health. Seafood, especially shellfish, commonly triggers allergic reactions. Wheat, corn, soy, nuts, milk, and eggs (especially the whites) cause their share of misery as well.

If you're allergic to a certain food you've eaten, you'll know—usually within 15 minutes. Your tongue will likely swell or itch, and you'll develop a rash on your skin. Other common symptoms include headache, stomach cramps, extreme flatulence, and diarrhea. Rarely, an allergic reaction may result in anaphylaxis, a potentially life-threatening condition in which blood pressure drops, the throat swells shut, and breathing becomes difficult.

True food allergies are actually quite rare. They affect less than 2 percent of the entire U.S. population. Most women who think they have food allergies more likely have a food intolerance.

If you have a food intolerance, you'll experience some of the same symptoms—namely headache and digestive upset. But food intolerance is never life-threatening. And you may be able to continue enjoying a problem food just by modifying how much or how often you eat it.

Only an allergist can say for sure whether you have a food allergy or a food intolerance. Get-make it through the five days. But when I finished the regimen, I was so happy I had stuck to it because I felt better than ever.

Then the nutritionist added one type of food back to my diet at a time. As soon as we added wheat, I got a sore throat. Wheat was the cause of all my problems!

Giving it up, though, wasn't so easy, and it wasn't long before I cheated. During Passover, I had to have matzo ball soup. The migraine came quickly. Still, I didn't believe that wheat could have such a powerful effect on my body. I stayed away from it for the next week or so until I was tempted by pizza. On came the migraine. I was finally convinced.

I've since found that eating a wheat-free diet is easy—at home. I can eat fruit, vegetables, fish, meats, eggs, nuts, and cheeses. I eat more rice, potatoes, and corn than ever before. And most health food stores carry pasta, cookies, crackers, and flour made from spelt, an ancient grain.

In the grocery store, I read labels like a detective—you never know where the wheat may be lurking. In restaurants, I make a point of avoiding things like sauces, cream soups, gravies, and meatballs, which may contain added wheat.

Life without wheat is challenging, but I feel great. In fact, it has launched me on a new career. I developed some delicious recipes for spelt crackers and cookies, and I'm selling to health food stores across the country.

---

ting an accurate diagnosis is critical, especially since a true allergy can be life-threatening.

If you're diagnosed with a food allergy, your doctor will likely advise you to steer clear of the offending food. These strategies can help you do just that.

**Scrutinize labels.** Food allergens routinely show up where you least expect them. For example, peanuts—which are responsible for more allergy-related deaths than any other food—go into pastries, breads, and meatballs. Even food additives such as emulsifiers and flavorings may contain peanuts. So before you buy any packaged food or beverage, carefully read the ingredient list.

**Be inquisitive.** When eating out, find out all you can about a dish before ordering it. Ask the server what ingredients are used and how it is prepared. If the server seems unsure, speak to the chef. Don't be shy—your health is at stake.

**Check cosmetics labels.** Believe it or not, cosmetics may contain food allergens. Milk, for example, is often used to make lipstick.

## Hay Fever

Hay fever has the dubious distinction of being the most common of all allergies.

The culprit is the pollen released by ragweed in autumn and certain grasses and trees in spring and summer. And while the sneezing, runny nose, headache, earache, sore throat, and watery eyes respond well to antihistamines, these medicines can make you tired. For hay fever relief without the drowsiness, try these measures.

**Get better with nettle.** An herb called stinging nettle can nip hay fever symptoms in the bud. Use freeze-dried nettle (available in health food stores) in capsules or teas. Try a small dose at first, since some people have a sensitivity to stinging nettle.

**Zero in on C.** In large doses, vitamin C acts as an antihistamine, but it doesn't work for everyone. If you want to try it, take 2,000 to 5,000 milligrams a day in divided doses.

*Note:* Some people develop diarrhea when taking more than 1,000 milligrams of vitamin C per day. If this happens to you, cut back your dosage until the diarrhea subsides.

**Be wary of melons.** If you are allergic to ragweed, you can get an itchy mouth when eating cantaloupe and other melons. If you're allergic to birch wood, you can get the same reaction when you eat apples or pears or drink chamomile tea. Doctors call this oral allergy syndrome. It isn't serious, but if you're bothered by an itchy mouth, steer clear of offending foods.

## Inhalant Allergies

Every day you breathe in as much as 2½ tablespoons of smoke, smog, car exhaust, and assorted other unsavory substances. For most of us, they drift by unnoticed. But if you have an inhalant allergy, certain airborne particles—especially pet dander, dust, and mold—can trigger an immune system response that mimics a respiratory infection. The usual symptoms include congestion; a runny, itchy nose; sneezing; and red, swollen eyes.

Inhalant allergies may be annoying, but unless you have asthma, they aren't life-threatening. Here's what to do to keep symptoms at bay.

**Snort salt water.** Add one-half teaspoon of salt and a pinch of baking soda to one cup of warm water. Allow the salt and baking soda to dissolve, then put the solution in a squeeze/spray bottle or a medicine dropper. Squirt the solution into one nostril, close the other, and sniff deeply. Switch nostrils and repeat to lubricate your sinuses and prevent sinus infection. You can do this three or four times a day.

**Get respite for sore eyes.** Run cool water over a clean washcloth. Lay the cloth over your eyes and leave it in place until it feels warm.

**Fight fire with fire.** Increase your consumption of hot and spicy foods such as ground red pepper, chili peppers, and hot-pepper sauce. The heat loosens mucus.

**Venture out after noon.** If your allergies are triggered by pollen and molds, stay indoors in the morning, when pollen and mold levels are at their highest.

**Clean house.** The goal is to get rid of dust mites, the microscopic bugs that feed on bits of shed skin and are well-known allergy aggravators. Their favorite hangout is in mattresses, so encase yours in a plastic cover and wash your bed linens in hot (130°F or warmer) water. And if you can, pull up your carpeting, which harbors dust mites, and live with hardwood, tile, or vinyl floors.

**Launder with eucalyptus oil.** Australian researchers found that laundering a wool blanket with eucalyptus oil slashed the dust mite population in the blanket by 95 percent. To begin, mix one part liquid dishwashing detergent

## ALLERGIES COME IN MANY GUISES

Allergic to eggs? Then put down that root beer!

This soda may owe its foamy mustache to the froth-producing alchemy of egg protein.

And unless you dissect the ingredients list, you won't know that troublesome peanuts could lurk in your barbecued spareribs (thickening the sauce) and that milk may be laced in your tuna fish. In fact, so-called dairy-free products may not be so far from the cow after all. (Nondairy creamers, for example, contain milk proteins.)

Labeling regulations still allow trace amounts of some ingredients to go unlisted, but for the most part, you can avoid surprise run-ins with your allergen by becoming a label sleuth. Use this list to become familiar with some of the less-than-obvious places where your allergen may show up.

| Food Source | Label Terms | Products to Check |
|---|---|---|
| Cow's milk | Calcium caseinate, casein hydrolysate, curds, lactalbumin, lactoglobulin, whey | Baked goods, egg substitute products, hot dogs, lunchmeats, nondairy creamers, snack foods, soups |
| Wheat | Farina, gluten, hydrogenated starch hydrolysates, semolina | Ale, beer, breakfast cereals, canned vegetables, gin, gravies, salad dressings, whiskey |
| Corn | Buretose, cerulose, dextrin, grits, hydrolyzed vegetable protein, lactic acid, sorbitol, vegetable gum, vegetable starch | Bourbon, breakfast cereals, juice, margarines, marshmallows, oils, snack foods, soft drinks, vinegar, vodka, wheat-based baked goods |
| Eggs | Albumin, egg powder, egg solids, globulin, ovalbumin, ovomucoid, ovovitellin | All baked goods, chocolate, coffee, ice cream, marshmallows, meat loaf, noodles, polenta, salad dressings, wines |
| Soy | Hydrolyzed vegetable protein, lecithin, soy flour, textured vegetable protein (TVP), tofu, vegetable gum, vegetable oil, vegetable starch | Breakfast cereals, canned soups, cheese substitutes, condiments, fast-food shakes, fried foods, margarine, meats, miso, tempeh, veggie burgers |
| Fish | Surimi | Imitation fish, sauces, soup stocks |
| Nuts | Hydrolyzed protein | Cookies and other baked goods, fried foods, gravies, sauces, vegetable oils |

For more comprehensive information on specific allergies, write to The Food Allergy Network, 10400 Eaton Place, Suite 107, Fairfax, VA 22030-2208.

(without bleach) in four parts eucalyptus oil. If the detergent doesn't dissolve the oil, try a different brand. Stir one teaspoon of the detergent-oil mixture into a glass of water. If the oil floats to the top within 10 minutes, it won't work. If it passes the test, mix one part detergent in four parts oil. Fill your washing machine with warm water, add the detergent-oil mixture, and then add your bedding. Let everything soak for 30 minutes, then finish the wash cycle.

# Good Digestion

Contrary to popular belief (and what your stomach seems to be telling you), digestive problems are not necessarily caused by something you ate.

"Certainly, food and nutrition are factors," says Kim Barrett, Ph.D., professor of medicine at the University of California, San Diego, School of Medicine. "But they're not solely to blame."

Some digestive ailments—like ulcers, for example—have ties to bacterial and viral infections. Others occur as side effects of medications, including antibiotics and prescription steroids. "There's also evidence that stress can aggravate conditions such as irritable bowel syndrome and inflammatory bowel disease, although we still don't understand why," says Dr. Barrett.

Another mystery is why women seem far more vulnerable to digestive problems than men are. Scientists think that hormonal fluctuations may play a role. "Women experience natural changes in their bowel habits during their monthly cycles, which would suggest some hormonal influence," notes Dr. Barrett.

What can you do to keep your digestive system healthy and minimize illness? First and foremost, build your meals and snacks around high-fiber, low-fat foods. And chew foods thoroughly. Saliva contains enzymes that help break down complex carbohydrates.

Exercise may also help digestion. "If your level of overall fitness improves, your digestive function will improve, too," Dr. Barrett says.

## Colitis

If you have colitis, which is an inflammation of the colon, we don't need to tell you how miserable it can be. A flare-up can cause abdominal pain, bloody stools, and diarrhea, sending you to bed with your misery.

No one seems to know why some people get colitis, but there's some indication that it could be related to stress. (Maybe this is why it's more of a woman's disease.) Medical research indicates that bacterial and parasitic infections such as salmonella can cause colitis. Also, temporary colitis can occur after taking certain types of antibiotics.

During flare-ups, you most likely can't avoid

taking prescription medicine. But along with it, try these natural strategies. They'll help reduce the symptoms and get you back on your feet faster.

**Favor bland fare.** Eat plain, low-fat, low-fiber foods such as dry toast, boiled skinless chicken, cooked carrots, and gelatin. These will treat your colon kindly.

**Avoid crunchy snacks.** Popcorn, nuts, and seeds can aggravate an already-angry colon. So steer clear until you're feeling better.

**Listen to your body.** If eating a certain food brings on pain, cross it off your menu.

**Emphasize fluids.** The diarrhea associated with colitis can leave you dehydrated. So drink at least 10 glasses of water or juice a day.

## Constipation

Some 18 million Americans frequently have problems moving their bowels—and two-thirds of them are women.

By and large, though, doctors blame constipation on poor nutrition—specifically, too many processed foods and too few fiber-rich foods such as grains, fruits, vegetables, and legumes. Ideally, you should be eating at least 25 grams of fiber a day. Yet most women consume just 12 grams a day, on average.

Preventing constipation can be as easy as gradually increasing your fiber intake. Work your way up to at least two servings of whole grains and five servings of fruits and vegetables each day. Some top-notch fiber sources include broccoli (2.3 grams per one-half cup), barley (2.9 grams per one-half cup), and raspberries (8 grams per one-half cup). High-fiber cereals provide even more—up to 11 grams or more per serving, depending on what you choose.

If you still become constipated from time to time, don't depend on chemically based laxatives to get things moving. These products can lead to

a condition called lazy bowel, in which you lose your ability to void naturally.

To restore regularity without risk, try these natural remedies.

**Sip apple juice.** Sorbitol, a natural sugar in apple juice, acts as a laxative. One glass of juice may be enough to stimulate a balky bowel.

**Go with the grain.** Mix one teaspoon of powdered psyllium seed or whole flaxseed in an eight-ounce glass of water or juice. Have this drink with each meal until your symptoms subside. Psyllium seed acts as a natural laxative, while flaxseed increases the bulk and water content of stool. (Because psyllium may inhibit the absorption of drugs, try to take it at least one hour after taking other medications.)

**Don't skip meals.** Eating stimulates food to move through the intestines. Breakfast is especially important because it gets your digestive juices flowing.

**Get your fill of water.** Constipation can be a sign that you're not drinking enough water. To keep your stools soft, aim for at least eight eight-ounce glasses a day.

**Hit the bricks.** Walking for 15 to 20 minutes a day stimulates bowel function, which supports regularity. Maintain a brisk pace—fast enough that talking is difficult but not impossible.

## Diarrhea

According to one study, women who have young children in day care are 10 to 25 percent more likely to develop diarrhea than women whose kids stay at home. The reason? Viruses and bacteria, including those that cause diarrhea, easily spread within groups of youngsters. And they pass the germs on to their moms.

But hand-to-mouth infections aren't the only cause of diarrhea. Loose, watery stools can result from consuming a food or beverage that you're sensitive to or that has spoiled. Caffeine, sorbitol (a sweetener added to diet sodas), antacids, antibiotics, and even stress can also contribute to diarrhea.

See your doctor if your diarrhea doesn't go away within 48 hours or if it's accompanied by other symptoms, such as fever, pain, or blood in the stool.

If your busy life has you on a strict timetable, try these natural remedies to speed relief.

**Soothe your intestines with tea.** Raspberry leaf contains tannins, substances that reduce intestinal inflammation. To make raspberry leaf tea, pour one cup of boiled water over two teaspoons of the herb. Steep for two to three minutes, then strain and allow to cool before drinking. You can buy raspberry leaf in health food stores.

**Get better with dried blueberries.** Dried blueberries contain inflammation-fighting tannins and pectin, a binding agent that helps solidify loose stools. Thoroughly chew and swallow three tablespoons of dried berries.

**Let slippery elm soothe you.** Slippery elm contains a substance that relieves intestinal irritation. Blend a few spoonfuls of slippery elm bark powder (sold in health food stores) with honey until you can roll the mixture into small balls. Dust the balls with more of the powder. When diarrhea strikes, let one ball slowly dissolve in your mouth. Repeat as necessary. Store leftover balls in a closed container in the refrigerator. (To keep the balls indefinitely, dry them in a very low oven—just the pilot light will work—for a few hours.)

**Eat light.** Consume only clear liquids such as chicken bouillon, herbal tea, and soft drinks (without artificial sweeteners or caffeine) for the first 24 hours after the onset of diarrhea. Then switch to small meals of bland foods such as bananas, rice, and crackers. Stick with this diet until you've been diarrhea-free for 24 hours, so your digestive tract has a chance to recuperate.

**Avoid dairy.** Eating dairy products while you have diarrhea can make you feel even worse because you temporarily lose your ability to digest lactose, a sugar in milk.

**Don't forget fluids.** Your body loses a lot of water when you have diarrhea. So drink at least 10 eight-ounce glasses of water a day.

## Food Poisoning

We all know the story of the picnic that went haywire because a well-meaning partier kept the mayo-based salad out in the sun too long. Sometimes a wedding makes the news because hundreds of guests end up in the emergency ward as a result of a less-than-careful caterer.

Yes, food poisoning is common. Millions of Americans contract some form of it each year. Sometimes, though rarely, it's fatal.

Food poisoning is totally preventable, so get familiar with the following advice.

- Set your refrigerator at 40°F or colder.
- Frequently wash your hands while preparing food, especially after handling raw meat, poultry, or fish and before handling other foods or utensils.
- Thoroughly clean the counter and cutting board after preparing food.
- Put away leftovers within two hours of finishing a meal (sooner in hot weather).

You'll end up with food poisoning if you consume food tainted with bacteria (such as *Escherichia coli* or salmonella) or a virus. These bugs usually populate raw or undercooked meats, poultry, and seafood; raw eggs; and unpasteurized dairy products and juices.

If your symptoms are extremely severe—you have bloody diarrhea and vomiting that cause dehydration—or they don't subside within four days, see a doctor. Usually, though, you can nurse yourself back to health with the following self-care measures.

**Defeat dehydration.** Mix one-half teaspoon of salt and three tablespoons of sugar in one quart of water. Drink one-half to one cup after each episode of diarrhea or 10 minutes after vomiting.

**Satisfy your thirst—and then some.** Diarrhea and vomiting rob your body of precious liquids. So drink plenty of water.

**Be kind to your digestive tract.** As your symptoms subside and you regain your appetite, very gradually reintroduce foods into your diet. Begin with broth, then add bland foods.

**Endure the diarrhea.** Don't take antidiarrheal medications while you have food poisoning. Diarrhea flushes bacteria out of your intestines.

## Gastritis

Gastritis is kind of like indigestion gone amok. It's a painful but rarely serious inflammation of the stomach lining.

While certain medications like aspirin or ibuprofen can cause gastritis, a bacteria called *Helicobacter pylori*, or *H. pylori*, is more often associated with it. Gastritis can either be silent or feel like an ulcer. The symptoms of both gastritis and ulcers are alike: abdominal pain, or burning below the breastbone. Only a doctor can determine if you have gastritis or a more serious condition.

For the prone, gastritis can attack when it's least expected. When it does happen, here's what to do.

**Choose calcium pills over milk.** Milk actually makes gastritis worse by triggering the release of stomach acid.

**Avoid the hot stuff.** While doctors no longer believe that spicy cuisine contributes to gastritis, patients still complain that it triggers an attack. Try cutting back or eliminating it entirely.

**Choose painkillers carefully.** Switch from aspirin or ibuprofen to acetaminophen to avoid stomach irritation.

**Keep antacids at hand.** Antacids almost always work at alleviating pain, so keep them handy in your purse. Don't take more than 16 antacid tablets daily. If your symptoms don't improve in two weeks, discontinue use and see your doctor.

## Heartburn

Every once in a while, stomach acid defies gravity. Rather than flowing south, it heads north into your esophagus. You feel pressure and a burning sensation beneath your breastbone, along with an acidic taste in your mouth. You have a classic case of heartburn—or, in medical terms, acid reflux.

While over-the-counter antacids remain the heartburn remedy of choice, you may not want to rely on drugs for relief. Fortunately, you have plenty of natural options.

Keep in mind, however, that many people who think they have heartburn are actually having heart pain. So don't take the symptoms lightly. If they don't go away within a few weeks, see your doctor. If the pain from your chest disperses to your shoulders, back, or neck or if it occurs while you're exercising, go to the emergency room immediately.

**Take a feet-first approach.** Standing up and moving around while you have heartburn helps clear acid from your esophagus. Avoid bending over or lying down, which can push your stomach acid back up.

**Watch the clock.** Avoid eating anything less than two hours before bedtime. Otherwise, the food reaches your stomach just as you're lying down, increasing the likelihood of stomach acid splashing into your esophagus.

**Skip the after-dinner mints.** Mint causes

## REAL-LIFE SCENARIO

### Her Food Choices Leave Her Burning

For years, Madeline and her husband have been celebrating the end of the work week with a casual Friday night dinner at the local Italian restaurant. She's wild about anchovies and hot peppers and always orders extras for her salad and pizza. She also treats herself to a few beers and an espresso. But ever since she turned 50, Madeline has added an extra "course" to her menu: Tums or Rolaids to try to counteract the uncomfortable burning sensation behind her breastbone that seems to splash into her throat. The discomfort wakes her up in the middle of the night, and her over-the-counter antacids don't seem to help. If she has to give up pizza, what's next?

That uncomfortable feeling Madeline is getting after dinner is most likely acid reflux, which simply means that stomach acid is creeping back up her esophagus when it should be busy breaking down her pizza and beer.

Madeline doesn't have to give up pizza or hot peppers, but she does need to cut back. Antacids can help relieve her symptoms, but they're not a cure. She should try cutting back on her Friday night fare until she gets to a level where the discomfort is gone. Also, because excess weight has been linked to heartburn, eating less will help Madeline drop a few pounds if she has a problem in that area.

Wearing loose, comfortable clothing will also help; Madeline shouldn't wear anything that's tight around the waist. Restrictive clothing encourages acid to go up instead of down. And to relieve discomfort at night, Madeline should stay seated upright for a while. Lying down or bending over also encourages stomach contents to churn upward instead of down.

At bedtime, Madeline should sleep on her back, with her head and chest elevated at a slant with a wedge or a phone book under her pillow. That should help keep her comfortably asleep while her stomach does its digestive work.

*Expert consulted*
*Melissa Palmer, M.D.*
*Gastroenterologist*
*Plainview, New York*

the gastroesophageal sphincter to relax, allowing stomach acid to back up into the esophagus. The same goes for coffee (even decaf) and chocolate.

**Delay post-meal workouts.** Wait at least an hour after a meal before exercising—all that movement promotes acid reflux.

## Irritable Bowel Syndrome

Irritable bowel syndrome (IBS) is sometimes confused with colitis. While the two conditions share many symptoms, they affect the digestive tract quite differently. In colitis, the intestinal lining becomes inflamed and ulcerated. In IBS, the lining twitches, spasms, and cramps uncontrollably.

If you have IBS, you probably experience episodes of abdominal pain, gas, constipation, or diarrhea—or a combination of all four symptoms. Some women's symptoms are so volatile that they alter their daily routines so they're always within range of a toilet.

While IBS can't be cured, you can reduce the frequency and severity of flare-ups with natural remedies. (All remedies mentioned are available in health food stores.) If they don't help, see your doctor.

**Counteract pain with cramp bark.** The herb cramp bark relaxes the muscular intestinal lining, easing the way for stool to exit the body. During a flare-up, take one to three capsules of cramp bark 15 minutes before each meal. Follow the label instructions for dosage.

**Go for the oil.** In a German study, 90 percent of people who took peppermint oil and caraway seed oil during a flare-up reported reductions in IBS pain. To try this remedy, add 5 to 10 drops of each oil to eight ounces of warm water. Drink before each meal.

*Note:* If you're pregnant, avoid caraway seed oil. It can harm a developing baby when taken in large doses. Also, taking peppermint oil for an extended time can cause serious stomach upset and inflammation.

**Take flaxseed by the spoonful.** Flaxseed oil is rich in eicosapentaenoic acid, an omega-3 fatty acid with anti-inflammatory properties. Drizzle two tablespoons of the oil onto your morning cereal daily. Or take it straight.

**Stir up a fiber supplement.** Make your own fiber supplement by combining one-quarter teaspoon powdered psyllium seed, one-quarter teaspoon whole flaxseed, and one-half teaspoon slippery elm bark powder in eight ounces of water. Then squeeze in the juice from a slice or two of lemon. Drink this two or three times a day for up to four days. It will work to move stool through your intestines.

**Profit from pectin.** Apple pectin, a granular supplement, is a good source of fiber. Sprinkle it on your food or dissolve it in liquid and drink it to supplement your daily fiber intake.

**Add spices later.** Season your food after it has been cooked. That way, the spices are less likely to irritate your digestive tract.

## Lactose Intolerance

If milk doesn't go down as easily as it used to, there's a good reason. As you get older, your intestines produce smaller and smaller amounts of the digestive enzyme lactase.

Lactase is necessary to break down lactose, a natural sugar found in milk and other dairy products. When your lactase levels decrease, you can become lactose intolerant. The symptoms—bloating, cramping, and diarrhea—can appear 15 minutes to several hours after you consume a dairy product.

Here's what you can do to better tolerate lactose intolerance.

**Cut your quantity.** Researchers at the University of Minnesota at St. Paul found that nearly everyone in a group of lactose-intolerant people could drink *one* eight-ounce glass of 2 percent milk a day without symptoms. By the way, all milk—fat-free, 1 percent, 2 percent, and whole—has the same amount of lactose.

**Choose yogurt over milk.** Yogurt containing active cultures has less lactose than most other dairy products. Read labels to find a brand with active cultures.

**Buy less lactose.** Some food manufacturers now offer lactose-free and lactose-reduced versions of milk and other dairy products.

**Watch for lactose in disguise.** Many foods are made with dairy products. Look for milk, cheese, or casein (a protein found in milk) among ingredients listed on canned foods, salad dressings, breads, and candy.

**Stretch your legs.** Walking for 30 minutes can ease bloating.

**Take a load off.** For stomach cramps, relaxing is a better remedy than staying active. Soak in a bath, prop up your feet, crawl into bed—whatever makes you feel better.

## Nausea and Vomiting

It begins as queasiness, a sickly sensation in the pit of your stomach. Sometimes the sensation passes without incident; other times it crescendos into full-fledged vomiting.

Nobody goes through life without encountering the totally depleting, wish-I-were-dead

## FOLK REMEDY: DOES IT WORK?

### Cola Syrup for Nausea

If you were a kid during the days when soda fountains were popular, chances are your mom bought you a sweet treat for an aching stomach: cola syrup.

"Cola syrup is thought to calm a queasy stomach because the concentrated sugars help relax the gastrointestinal tract," explains Melanie Cupp, Pharm.D., drug information specialist at the West Virginia University School of Pharmacy in Morgantown. "It can actually calm a queasy stomach within minutes. Pregnant women swear by it for relieving morning sickness."

Just because corner soda fountains are hard to come by these days doesn't mean this folk remedy must disappear. Cola syrup can be bought without a prescription at your neighborhood pharmacy. Just ask your pharmacist.

Cola syrup will lose its ability to relax the stomach if diluted. For this reason, other liquids should not be consumed for at least 15 minutes after taking a dose. No more than five doses (one to two tablespoons each) should be taken within one hour; otherwise, stomach pain and diarrhea may occur, explains Dr. Cupp.

**RECOMMENDATION:** Worth a Try

apparent reason or after receiving new medication, see your doctor.

**Suck on ginger candy.** For any type of nausea, ginger is said to work as well as the over-the-counter medicine dimenhydrinate (Dramamine). When you start feeling queasy, suck on crystallized ginger-root candy. It's sold in health food stores and gourmet food shops.

**Sip a glass of ginger ale.** Ginger ale contains enough real ginger to subdue mild nausea.

**Keep crackers handy.** Nibbling on crackers helps take the edge off nausea. Just stick with small portions.

**Get fluids going.** If you vomit, don't eat anything for a couple of hours afterward, so your stomach has an opportunity to settle down. Then start sipping fluids such as water, flat soda, sports drinks, and chicken broth.

## Stomachache

When a stomachache strikes, you'll experience pain, cramping, and possibly constipation or diarrhea. An upset stomach usually goes away on its own within 24 hours. For faster relief, try these stomach-soothing remedies. (If your symptoms don't subside within a few days or if they are severe and a fever or bloody stool accompanies them, see your doctor to rule out colitis, an ulcer, food poisoning, or other serious stomach conditions.)

**Turn to herbs.** Drink a cup of chamomile or peppermint tea three or four times a day until you feel better. Both of these herbs gently relieve stomach upset. You can buy herbal teas in health food stores and supermarkets.

experience of nausea and vomiting. Women who've had children are all too familiar with it: Morning sickness is common in the initial stages of pregnancy. (You'll find this addressed in Easing Childbirth and Recovery on page 138.)

Ironically, as bad as vomiting makes you feel, it's sometimes good for you. Nausea and vomiting are often the result of something bad in your body that your body wants to get rid of. If this is the case, let it do its job.

If you continue to feel sick for more than three days or experience frequent nausea for no

*Note:* Chamomile can cause an allergic reaction, but it's rare. If you are allergic to related plants such as asters, chrysanthemums, and ragweed, take caution when drinking the tea.

If you have stomach cramps, try peppermint oil capsules, which also are available in health food stores. Take one capsule two or three times a day between meals until you feel relief.

*Note:* During pregnancy, women should never take peppermint because it could harm the fetus.

**Eat less more often.** Small, frequent meals are easier on your stomach than the standard three squares. So during the day, eat mini-meals of bland foods.

**Take a breather.** When you're stressed, deep breathing can stop your stomach from churning. Sit in a straight-back chair and slowly inhale, feeling your abdomen expand. Then slowly exhale, feeling your diaphragm (the muscle that separates your chest and abdomen) relax.

**Hit the spot with heat.** Lie down and place a hot-water bottle wrapped in a thin towel across your stomach. The heat can relax a knotted stomach or abdominal muscle and relieve pain.

**Slurp soup.** Experts can't yet explain why exactly, but chicken soup is a bland food that helps cleanse the digestive tract and relax stomach cramps.

**Sip warm ginger ale.** Take frequent small sips. Ginger stimulates the production of saliva, which neutralizes stomach acid.

**Chew gum.** Like ginger ale, chewing gum gets saliva flowing. Chew for 30 minutes at the onset of an upset stomach or heartburn. Avoid gum with artificial sweeteners, which can have a laxative effect.

**Loosen your belt.** Clothes that fit tightly around your waist put pressure on your stomach.

## Ulcers

Although ulcers have long had a reputation as a "guy problem," women get them just as often as men. But while men are more likely to develop duodenal ulcers (in the upper segment of the small intestine), women are more susceptible to gastric ulcers (in the stomach).

You've also probably heard that ulcers are

---

**FOLK REMEDY: DOES IT WORK?**

### Milk for Ulcers

There was a time when milk was a liquid security blanket, a cure-all comfort food. Our midnight friend lulled us to rest when we couldn't bear counting one more sheep; along with cookies, it dried up tears after a tricycle fall; and during an ulcer flare-up, it seemed like the only thing that would bring soothing relief.

"If milk works, it's probably psychological," says Susan Calvert Finn, R.D., Ph.D., director of nutrition at Roth Laboratories in Columbus, Ohio, and author of *The American Dietetic Association Guide to Women's Nutrition for Healthy Living*.

It's understandable why people with ulcerated innards historically reached for milk. The high alkalinity of dairy products can be soothing for some people, says Dr. Finn. Yet, because it's a protein, milk is not easy to digest. In fact, dairy products require high secretions of nothing other than stomach acid. (So the hearty job of processing milk can keep you up at night, meaning it fails as an insomnia cure, too.)

**RECOMMENDATION: Forget It**

caused by acidic foods, excessive alcohol consumption, smoking, or stress—and they are. But research now shows that many ulcers can be linked to the spiral-shaped *Helicobacter pylori* bacteria.

Researchers suspect that *H. pylori* do their damage by penetrating and weakening the digestive tract's protective lining, making it more vulnerable to stomach acids.

If you have an ulcer caused by this bacterium, your doctor will likely put you on a course of antibiotics along with medications to suppress gastric acid. In 90 percent of cases, *H. pylori* ulcers treated with antibiotics never return.

Not every ulcer results from *H. pylori*, however. Some are due to excessive use of aspirin and other nonsteroidal anti-inflammatory drugs, including ibuprofen.

No matter what the cause of your ulcer, a few simple strategies help control the gnawing, burning pain and quicken the healing process.

**Steer clear of caffeine and citrus.** While experts no longer believe that specific foods cause ulcers, coffee and citrus fruits and juices are known to worsen ulcer symptoms.

**Avoid aspirin and ibuprofen.** They're bad news for ulcer-prone stomachs. Instead, take acetaminophen for aches, pains, or headaches.

**Drink cabbage juice.** Historically, cabbage has had such a good track record for healing ulcers that at one time it was suspected to contain a new vitamin—vitamin U. Scientists now know that cabbage's anti-ulcer power comes from an amino acid that stimulates the mucous membrane in the stomach to thicken. Deep healing results as the pits in your digestive lining close over.

Drinking about a liter a day (about one quart) for three weeks has yielded these heroic results.

Fresh is certainly best, but if you don't have a juicer, cabbage juice can be found at health food stores, sometimes under the guise of sauerkraut juice. (Mixing cabbage with other vegetable or fruit juices may help improve the taste.) You can also munch on half a head of cabbage throughout the day.

**Have a little honey.** This golden medicine was specifically prescribed by Middle Eastern and Russian folk healers to cure ulcers long before bacteria was determined to be the cause. Modern science now qualifies honey's tremendous antibacterial properties, validating yet another bit of folk wisdom.

**Get a little culture.** Acidophilus and lactobacillus are among the friendly bacteria found in cultured food. The more of these good guys you have populating your stomach lining, the less room there is for bully bacteria *H. pylori* to move in and nibble away at your stomach lining.

If you are already taking antibiotics for *H. pylori*, supplement them with one cup of yogurt three or four times daily.

**Feed your ulcer fiber.** Since ulcer pain can roar back when your stomach growls, try to keep your inner animal sated on a standard feeding schedule. Try to get 35 grams of fiber each day by loading up on fruits, vegetables, and whole grains.

**Put some spice in your life.** Cayenne pepper can stimulate blood flow to the stomach, which activates healing. Ingest a small capsule of powdered cayenne pepper, or sip red pepper tea with one-quarter teaspoon of cayenne pepper steeped in one cup of hot water. You can drink this tea on a daily basis to help prevent the recurrence of ulcers. Modern medicine also has shown that pepper has a mild anesthetic effect.

# Your Healthy Heart

**Y**our heart beats 100,000 times a day, sending some 2,000 gallons of life-sustaining blood coursing through 60,000 miles of blood vessels. So you can appreciate why taking good care of your heart is so important. The healthier it is, the more efficiently it will function—and the longer it will keep you kicking.

Unfortunately, heart disease remains the number one cause of death among American women, surpassing even breast cancer. According to Alice H. Lichtenstein, D.Sc., professor of nutrition at the Jean Mayer USDA Human Nutrition Research Center on Aging at Tufts University in Boston, one in two women will die from heart disease, while one in eight will die from breast cancer.

Thanks to the hormone estrogen, women rarely develop heart disease as early in adulthood as men. Estrogen helps keep women's arteries clear and healthy by regulating the amounts of low-density lipoprotein (LDL) cholesterol, the bad kind that clogs, and high-density lipoprotein (HDL) cholesterol, the good kind that escorts LDL from your body.

Estrogen's protective effects diminish at menopause, however, as the body's production of the hormone declines. At menopause, a woman's risk of heart disease begins to climb, and by the time she reaches age 65, it's about equal to a man's. Despite these odds, women tend to pay less attention to heart health than they should. "Some women simply aren't aware of their risk," Dr. Lichtenstein notes. "Other women are aware, but they're not as concerned about it as they are about breast cancer."

Doctors are eager to spread the word that a woman can do a lot to reduce her chances of getting heart disease in the first place. In this chapter, they share their best advice for minimizing major risk factors—including angina, high blood pressure, and high cholesterol—and offer tips for keeping your heart healthy.

## Prevention Is So Simple

Some risk factors for heart disease—such as age, race, and family history—you cannot change. That said, there's still plenty that you can do to prevent heart disease (and even reverse existing damage).

### REAL-LIFE SCENARIO

#### She's Putting Her Heart at Risk

**Katherine knows she's at risk for heart disease. She smokes too much (even though she has quit three times) and doesn't exercise much, and her job as a receptionist for a law firm keeps her at her desk all day. As she approaches her 50th birthday, she's very aware of the fact that her father died of a heart attack at that age. But Katherine is doing what she can to protect herself. She takes megadoses of vitamin C to offset the effects of smoking. Because she's slim and doesn't gain weight, she thinks that she doesn't have to exercise. And she loves garlic, which she's heard is a big heart protector, so she eats it every chance she gets. How "safe" is Katherine when it comes to risk of heart disease?**

Not as safe as she thinks.

Katherine has at least four risk factors for heart disease: family history of disease, lack of exercise, cigarette smoking, and the fact that she's approaching menopause, which means that she'll be losing a lot of the heart-protecting hormone estrogen. So her birthday present to herself should be a visit to her doctor for a complete physical examination. She may have other risk factors that she doesn't know about, such as high blood pressure or high cholesterol, which only a physical will uncover.

As Katherine blows out the candles on her cake, she should vow to make a healthy heart her priority. Natural remedies such as vitamin C and garlic may complement healthy living, but the fact remains that no amount of vitamins or dietary changes is going to offset the effects of smoking and a sedentary lifestyle. Katherine needs to get help for her tobacco addiction, and she has to start exercising. Exercise is important to a woman's heart health, no matter what her weight.

*Expert consulted*
*Cheryl Martin, M.D.*
*Cardiologist and assistant clinical professor of*
*cardiovascular medicine*
*Milwaukee Heart Institute*

**Snuff the butts.** For women, smoking stands head and shoulders above all other risk factors for heart disease. A woman who smokes is two to six times more likely to experience a heart attack than a woman who has never smoked. Almost all women who have heart attacks before age 50 are smokers.

**Slim down.** Carrying a little extra body fat is okay as long as it's settled on your hips, thighs, and backside. But if you are more than 20 percent above your ideal weight or if fat has taken up residence around your waist, your risk for heart disease edges upward.

To quickly calculate your ideal weight, use this simple formula, known as the body mass index (BMI), a ratio of weight to height. Divide your weight (in pounds) by your height (in inches) squared. Multiply the resulting number by 705 to get your BMI.

A woman who weighs 145 pounds and is five feet, four inches tall (64 inches), for example, would divide 145 by 4,096 (her height in inches squared) to get 0.0354, which she would then multiply by 705. The answer rounds up to 25 and represents her BMI.

Doctors say that a healthy BMI is somewhere between 19 and 24. One large-scale study points to a BMI below 21 as ideal for preventing heart disease in women.

**Be frugal with fat.** Saturated dietary fat accelerates the progression of heart disease. Doctors recommend limiting your total daily fat intake to 30 percent of calories, with no more than 7 percent of those calories coming from saturated fat. To help achieve this without doing a lot of arithmetic, limit yourself to no more than six ounces of lean meat, fish, or poultry a day and use skim and low-fat dairy products.

**Use olive oil in place of other fats.** Olive oil consists mostly of monounsaturated fatty acids, which have been shown to lower LDL cholesterol levels while raising HDL levels. But don't go overboard; oil is still 100 percent fat.

**Fill up with fiber.** By substituting high-fiber foods for high-fat ones, you'll decrease your LDL cholesterol. Add oat bran, oatmeal, barley, and beans to your menus for a good dose of soluble fiber, the type that researchers say is especially effective.

**Make produce your pal.** Build your meals around a variety of foods, including plenty of antioxidant-rich fruits and vegetables. Antioxidants—vitamins C and E and beta-carotene—neutralize highly destructive molecules called free radicals. In this way, the nutrients defend artery walls against the damage that triggers plaque accumulation. Eat at least five servings of antioxidant-rich fruits and vegetables, including broccoli, carrots, collard greens, Swiss chard, citrus fruits, papaya, and cantaloupe, each day.

**Include tomatoes, too.** Tomatoes are the best source of lycopene, a compound that appears to protect against heart disease. Just one-half cup of tomato sauce supplies 22 milligrams, three-quarters cup of tomato juice has 20 milligrams, and one-half cup of chopped fresh tomatoes supplies 8 milligrams.

**Give garlic the green light.** Garlic contains allicin, a compound that appears to lower cholesterol and blood pressure. Eat one clove a day, using chopped, fresh garlic to flavor salads and cooked dishes.

**Sip a little wine (or grape juice).** Compounds known as flavonoids may prevent LDL cholesterol from sticking to artery walls and may stop blood platelets from clumping together and forming dangerous clots. Flavonoids are found in abundance in red wine and grape juice. Other sources include onions, apples, broccoli, and tea. If you choose to drink red wine, keep in mind that studies have shown that moderate alcohol consumption—just one drink a day—increases breast cancer risk by 30 to 40 percent. If you have a family history of breast cancer, restrict yourself to two or three drinks a week. A drink equals five ounces of wine.

**Invest in supplemental insurance.** Even if you eat healthfully, you may not get enough of certain nutrients to protect against heart disease. A multivitamin/mineral supplement can cover any deficit. Make sure that your multivitamin contains vitamin $B_6$, vitamin $B_{12}$, and folate. These nutrients help prevent the chemical changes that lead to atherosclerosis (hardening and clogging of the arteries).

**Do some legwork.** Make sure you do a minimum of 30 minutes of heart-pumping aerobic activity (such as brisk walking, running, or cycling) three or four times a week. Aerobic exercise strengthens and tones your heart muscle, so your heart pumps more blood with each beat. And it reduces the stickiness of platelets, making them less likely to form clots.

**Control diabetes.** Diabetes can increase your risk for heart disease fourfold. If you have diabetes, work with your doctor to develop a diet, exercise, and weight-loss program geared toward monitoring and managing your blood sugar levels.

## Angina

The recurring pressure in your chest has you wondering whether you're experiencing the first

## KNOW YOUR NUMBERS

It's all about numbers. Your blood pressure readings and cholesterol and triglyceride levels (along with diet and exercise patterns, smoking, and heredity) determine your risk for heart disease. This is one case where ignorance is not bliss. Take a look at the numbers below, which are the guidelines used by researchers from the Framingham Heart Study, and then have yourself checked.

### Blood Pressure (mm. Hg)

| Rating | Systolic (top no.) | Diastolic (bottom no.) |
|---|---|---|
| Ideal | 120 or lower | 80 or lower |
| Normal | 129 or lower | 84 or lower |
| High Normal | 130–139 | 85–89 |
| Mild Hypertension | 140–159 | 90–99 |
| Moderate Hypertension | 160–179 | 100–109 |
| Severe Hypertension | 180 or higher | 110 or higher |

### Cholesterol (mg./dl.)

| Rating | LDL | HDL | Total |
|---|---|---|---|
| Desirable | 130 or lower | 45 or higher | 150 or lower |
| Borderline High | 131–159 | — | 151–239 |
| High | 160 or higher | — | 240 or higher |

### Triglycerides (mg./dl.)

| Rating | Total |
|---|---|
| Desirable | 150 or lower |
| Normal | 200 or lower |
| Borderline High | 200–400 |
| High | 400–1,000 |
| Very High | 1,000 or higher |

signs of heart trouble. You're wise to wonder, because angina is a warning sign that should never be ignored.

Angina occurs when your heart isn't getting enough oxygen-rich blood. The resulting pain—usually in your chest but sometimes in your jaw or arm—subsides once your heart's oxygen needs are met.

As it turns out, not everyone who has angina eventually experiences a heart attack (when blood flow to the heart becomes completely blocked). In fact, angina seems less likely to lead to heart attacks in women than in men.

If you have angina, your doctor will most likely prescribe nitroglycerin, a medication that dilates the heart's arteries. Follow her instructions carefully when using this medication. In addition, try the following strategies to minimize angina pain and discourage future attacks.

**Stop what you are doing.** When you feel an angina attack coming on, sit down and rest. If you have clogged arteries, this reduces the workload on your heart and alleviates pain.

**Thwart attacks with hawthorn.** Research has shown that the herb hawthorn contains substances that open arteries and improve blood flow to the heart. Naturopathic doctors recommend taking 240 to 480 milligrams of standardized hawthorn extract each day. While hawthorn is natural, it is a powerful medicine, so do not take it without first discussing it with your doctor.

## High Blood Pressure

It doesn't hurt and it has no symptoms, yet one out of every four women between the ages of 35 and 55, and one of every two women over age 55, has high blood pressure. Most don't even know it.

Doctors define high blood pressure as a consistent reading of 140/90 mm. Hg (millimeters of mercury) or higher. A reading that is 120/80 mm. Hg is considered ideal.

High blood pressure is as mysterious as it is silent. Scientists don't know why some of us get high blood pressure, but they do know that certain factors contribute to a woman's vulnerability.

- Ethnic background—African-American, Puerto Rican, Cuban, or Mexican
- Overweight
- Birth control pills
- Stress
- Diabetes or a disease that affects the kidneys, adrenal glands, or other glands

High blood pressure is potentially dangerous because it stresses the arteries, putting you at risk for heart attack and stroke. Left untreated, it can also lead to kidney failure.

Medication can help control high blood pressure, helping to prevent its potential damage. If you can't get it under control using natural methods, your doctor may prescribe medication.

### LOW BLOOD PRESSURE: WOMEN'S LUCK?

The scenario: As you get up to leave your doctor's office, she informs you that your blood pressure reading was only 80/60. You faint.

Why? Because (a) you panicked because you think that "normal" blood pressure is closer to 120/80; (b) you stood up too fast; (c) it was that lumberjack breakfast you ate; (d) you're overjoyed because it will help you live longer.

The answer: D.

Thanks to the female hormone estrogen, women often have lower blood pressure readings than men. It's only when your typical reading drops significantly that something might be wrong.

So instead of writing you a prescription, your doctor congratulates you.

"Low blood pressure puts you at lower risk for cardiovascular disease, stroke, and kidney disease. It's usually something to be glad about," says Clarita E. Herrera, M.D., clinical instructor in primary care at the New York Medical College in Valhalla, New York, and attending physician at Lenox Hill Hospital in New York City.

The only problem with hypotension is that it can make you lightheaded when you move your body quickly. The key is to be are aware of this and train yourself to move mindfully, Dr. Herrera says. When you're getting out of bed, for example, pause in a seated position and take a few deep breaths.

Also keep in mind that as levels of protective estrogen decline during menopause, your blood pressure could start going up (as does your risk for heart disease). Be sure to have it checked regularly.

But nondrug options like the following can knock points off your reading, too. (If you are already taking blood pressure medication, be sure to consult your doctor before making any changes in your dosage.)

**Savor the "stinking rose."** Studies show that allicin, the compound in garlic that helps lower cholesterol, reduces blood pressure as well. The suggested intake is one clove per day.

**Tap the power of potassium.** In one study, a daily 3,120-milligram dose of potassium slashed an average of seven points from participants' systolic blood pressures (the top number in a reading). Their diastolic pressures (the bottom number) also dropped an average of two points. Good food sources of potassium include baked potatoes, cantaloupe, and spinach. Other potassium-rich foods include bananas, beans, honeydew, orange juice, prunes, and raisins. Aim for an intake of 2,000 to 4,000 milligrams a day.

**Count up calcium.** At least two studies have found that moms-to-be who take supplemental calcium reduce their chances of developing pregnancy-related high blood pressure. If you're pregnant or nursing, you need 1,200 to 1,500 milligrams of calcium a day.

**Check out coenzyme $Q_{10}$ and l-carnitine.** When taken together, coenzyme $Q_{10}$ (an antioxidant) and l-carnitine (an amino acid) may help lower blood pressure and strengthen heart muscle contractions. Both supplements are sold in health food stores.

**Salt sensibly.** Salt is not the cardiovascular villain it was once thought to be. In fact, some research suggests that consuming up to 4,000 milligrams of sodium a day won't necessarily raise your blood pressure, as long as you're also taking in enough magnesium and potassium. Still, you're wise to use salt judiciously. Limit yourself to one teaspoon (2,000 milligrams) a day.

**Crunch celery.** Thanks to its mild diuretic properties, celery may help lower blood pressure by reducing the amount of fluid in the bloodstream. Eat at least four stalks a day.

## High Cholesterol

With all we've heard about the dangers of cholesterol, you'd think that it's something we could gladly do without. The truth is, though, that we can't live without cholesterol. It's only when levels get too high that we have to do something about it.

What constitutes "high" is also up for debate. Some researchers say that to be completely on the safe side, your total cholesterol reading should be under 150 mg./dl. (milligrams per deciliter), which is difficult for some people to achieve. More commonly, we're told that a total reading of 240 mg./dl. is the safe limit.

More recently, researchers have been finding that it's not total cholesterol at all but the ratio between good HDL and bad LDL that's the leading indicator. The total doesn't matter as long as your LDL is no higher than 130 and your HDL is 45 or higher. And the higher your HDL, the better.

This means that if your total comes out on the high side, you don't need to panic. Ask your doctor to take readings for HDL and LDL. If it still doesn't look good, practice the prevention techniques mentioned above. Plus, you can try the following home remedies that studies have shown can help reduce cholesterol.

**Befriend fenugreek.** In one study, participants who consumed three-quarters cup of the herb fenugreek every day for 20 days cut their LDL levels by one-third. (Their HDL levels stayed the same.) Eat one to two tablespoons of ground fenugreek seeds three or four times a day. If you don't like the taste of the seeds, you can take one or two 580-milligram capsules three or four times a day. Both ground seeds and capsules are sold in most health food stores.

**Try turmeric.** Turmeric, a staple of Indian cuisine, enhances the body's ability to process cholesterol. Sprinkle the ground herb on poultry, fish, and beans. Or take 150 milligrams in capsule form (available in most health food stores) three times a day.

**Make it hot, hot, hot.** Hot peppers contain capsaicin, an oil that can keep LDL cholesterol from sticking to artery walls.

**Go fishin'.** Certain species of fish—including mackerel, salmon, and tuna—are rich in omega-3 fatty acids. Omega-3's may lower heart-harming LDL while sustaining heart-healthy HDL. Eat at least one three-ounce serving of omega-3–rich fish per week.

**Enjoy soy.** Soy contains phytoestrogens, compounds that shuttle LDL from the bloodstream to the liver, where it's broken down and excreted. Choose from an array of soy products and aim for 20 to 25 grams of soy protein a day.

**Get the flax.** Studies have shown that flaxseed lowers LDL while preserving HDL, probably because of its high fiber content. Look for ground flaxseed in health food stores. Sprinkle a tablespoon or more on hot or cold cereal, soup, or yogurt.

**Consider C.** In one study, people with low vitamin C levels who took 1,000 milligrams of the nutrient every day for eight months raised their HDL readings by 7 percent, on average.

# Pain, Pain Gone Away

This may come as little comfort when you slip a disk moving the sofa or break a bone running down the steps, but pain is good. Imagine what would happen if you kept running on a broken foot!

Pain comes in two varieties. Acute pain, the kind you get when you bang your knee, comes on suddenly and goes away when the injury is gone. All of us have had it, and we're sure to have it again. It can last for anywhere from a few minutes to a few weeks. A little rest, maybe some ice at first or heat later, and over-the-counter pain relievers are usually enough to get you through it.

The other kind of pain, chronic pain, is more insidious. Some injuries and diseases create pain that lingers on and off for months and sometimes years. It's estimated that more than 67 million people in the United States experience chronic pain.

In this chapter, you'll find natural relief for some of the most common causes of acute and chronic pain. If you have already been diagnosed with a problem and are taking medication for it, do not discontinue your medication without consulting with your doctor. If you have pain that's associated with a disease such as lupus or arthritis, or if you have unexplained or unbearable pain, you should see your doctor to find out the cause, cautions Margaret Caudill, M.D., Ph.D., co-director of the department of pain medicine at Dartmouth Hitchcock Clinic in Manchester, New Hampshire, and author of *Managing Pain Before It Manages You.*

## Arthritis

If you're over age 45, it's likely that you've already experienced arthritis pain. If not, you surely will by the time you retire, even if it's just a twinge in the knee.

But arthritis isn't just the purview of the aging. In one survey of 24,000 women, nearly 9 percent of those between ages 15 and 44 said that they had arthritis pain.

Researchers have identified more than 100 forms of arthritis. The two most common—and the ones that affect women the most—are osteoarthritis and rheumatoid arthritis.

Osteoarthritis is caused by the gradual breakdown of cartilage, the soft, spongy material that cushions joints. It can also result from injury—that skating accident you had as a kid can show up decades later as arthritis. Overweight is a factor, too.

Rheumatoid arthritis is considered a younger person's pain. It affects mostly women in their thirties, forties, and fifties. Medically speaking, it's classified as an autoimmune disease. In other words, the body's immune system turns on itself—in this case, causing the synovial membrane, which lubricates each joint, to become inflamed.

For either type of arthritis, many doctors recommend nonsteroidal anti-inflammatory drugs to minimize pain, swelling, and stiffness. The following nondrug remedies can also ease discomfort and improve joint mobility.

**Give peas a chance.** Wrap a bag of frozen peas in a towel and apply it to the swollen joint for 10 to 15 minutes, two or three times a day. The cold reduces inflammation.

**Create a rice pack.** To warm painful stiff joints, fill a soft white tube sock with five to eight inches of uncooked rice. Knot the sock or tie it shut with string. Heat it in the microwave for two minutes, then check the temperature before applying it to the affected joint. If you can comfortably hold the sock, it's not too hot. Rest the pack on the affected area and leave it in place until it cools down. The heat increases blood circulation, which in turn helps loosen and soothe the area.

## WOMAN TO WOMAN
### She Uses Exercise to Overcome Pain

*Kathy Hammons of Rolling Meadows, Illinois, was diagnosed with debilitating rheumatoid arthritis at age 26. Over the next 14 years, she fought her way through pain and surgery by doing what she loves best: exercising. Today an aerobics teacher and personal trainer, she's teaching others like her how to overcome arthritis through movement.*

I have always been an active person. In fact, I was juggling two full-time jobs—teaching aerobics classes and working as a bartender and waitress—when I first started experiencing the symptoms of what turned out to be rheumatoid arthritis.

It started with stiffness and pain in my hands that made it hard to lift trays of food. To think that this was happening to me, someone so physically fit!

It hit me fast. Over the next decade, I had several surgeries on my hands to repair and replace deteriorated tendons. I lost some mobility in my fingers, and I now have to wear hand splints at night to help keep my tendons from tightening while I sleep. The arthritis has attacked the joints in my feet, too, and is starting to move into my shoulder and jaw.

Through all the pain and operations, I never gave up on exercise. It has made the difference in my life. As unlikely as it must sound, I found that exercise actually helped me deal with the pain. In fact, it's now my one and only full-time job.

Because of what I went through, I wanted to show others how important it is to be physically active when you have a debilitating disease. I'm still teaching exercise classes, only now, some of them are for people with arthritis. I teach them how to regain mobility, and together, we remain fit.

We work in a very warm therapy pool, where the warmth helps our joints feel better, and the water helps support our bodies so that we move more easily and don't feel the full impact of our weight on our joints. Very slowly and gently, we stretch and tone our bodies from head to toe.

Although I have had to change a lot of things in my life, arthritis has taught me an important lesson: how to listen to my body, test my limits, and live a happy life within those limits.

**Reach for the chile.** If you have osteoarthritis, try an over-the-counter cream made with capsaicin, a chile pepper extract, such as Capzasin or Arthricare. It depletes a chemical in the nerves, called substance P, that sends pain messages to the brain.

**Check out curcumin.** For rheumatoid arthritis, take 400 milligrams of curcumin three times a day until the flare-up subsides. Curcumin, the yellow pigment in turmeric, can relieve swelling and improve joint mobility. Curcumin capsules are available in health food stores.

**Eat your fish.** Certain species of fish, including Atlantic herring and Atlantic salmon, contain omega-3 fatty acids. Omega-3's have been shown to reduce the inflammation of rheumatoid arthritis. Eat at least one three-ounce serving of omega-3–rich fish each day.

**Keep joints moving.** While it may seem impossible when you're hurting, exercise can actually reduce pain. Regular low-impact aerobic exercise such as swimming and riding an exercise bicycle increases the circulation of fluid around joints and strengthens the muscles that support joints. Avoid exercise if your joints are red, hot, and swollen, though.

## Back Pain

It's almost as common as the common cold, but back pain lingers much longer. In fact, it's responsible for about six million doctor visits a year, many of them from women who spend all day sitting in front of computers.

Most back pain goes away on its own within a few days to a week. But if you don't want to wait it out, these self-care measures can help. If

> ### REAL-LIFE SCENARIO
> #### Her Back Is Keeping Her Down
>
> **At only 42 years of age, Denise is threatened with excruciating pain every time she uses her back. She threw her back out a few years ago trying to move the refrigerator to clean and landed in bed for a week. Ever since, she has had repeated episodes of pain and is losing more and more time from work. She has been the chiropractor route, but spinal adjustments produce only temporary relief. And she's tired of going back again and again. She's resisting seeing an orthopedic surgeon, fearing that the doctor will only recommend surgery. She's at the point where she feels that there are no other options. Is surgery her only salvation?**
>
> **D**enise's muscle strength has probably declined as she's gotten older, especially if she's had children and has been carrying them around for years. So when she lifts or moves something heavy, she strains her weakened back muscles and ends up in pain.
>
> Denise's visit to the chiropractor helped realign the joints in her spine that got out of place, but the adjustments did

these remedies don't help or if the pain is so great that you can't tolerate it, then see your doctor.

**Hold it right there.** When back pain strikes, stop what you're doing. The pain is your body's way of telling you that you're doing something the wrong way. Try to figure out what's wrong and make adjustments. Perhaps you can then continue the activity in comfort.

**Get help from heat.** For back pain caused by a muscle spasm, soak a washcloth in comfortably hot water and place it over the affected area. Resoak the cloth every 3 minutes or so to keep it warm. Continue the applications for up to 30 minutes.

**Try ice.** To relieve a back injury within the first 24 hours, apply a towel-wrapped ice pack to little to prevent it from happening again. That's because the adjustments did nothing to strengthen the muscles that are responsible for pulling her back out of alignment in the first place. But she does have another option: physical therapy.

A physical therapist can help Denise learn both strengthening and flexibility, or stretching, exercises that will retrain her posture, keep her lower back stable, and strengthen her abdominal muscles, which support the lower back. Then Denise needs to continue these exercises on her own to prevent further trouble.

It's probably a good idea for Denise to see a doctor, too. After all this time, it's possible that arthritis could be developing in the small joints of her spine, which could also be contributing to the pain. Or she could have a ruptured disk. But she needn't fear. Both conditions can be treated medically—without surgery.

*Expert consulted*
*Kathryn Stolp-Smith, M.D.*
*Physiatrist*
*Mayo Clinic*
*Rochester, Minnesota*

the affected area for 5 to 10 minutes. Repeat every hour.

**Take it lying down.** For lower-back pain, lie on the floor with a pillow positioned under your knees so that they bend slightly. This rests your iliopsoas muscles, which extend from your lower back around either side of your body to the thighbone.

**Stop pain by stretching.** Stop pain before it starts by relieving tightness and stiffness in your back. Stand in front of a table and bend forward so that you can rest your torso on the table. Your torso should form a 90-degree angle with your thighs. Extend your arms in front of you, then breathe slowly as you bend your knees slightly. Hold for two minutes, then brace yourself with your arms and stand up straight.

**Move soon.** Don't let an aching back keep you in bed for more than two days. After 48 hours of bed rest, your circulation slows down, your muscles and joints stiffen, and your back pain gets worse.

## Chronic Pain

You may or may not know what causes it. But it doesn't really matter—all you know is that it doesn't go away. Chronic pain is debilitating, and it can affect more than your health. It can cause a dramatic change in your lifestyle and in your relationships with family and friends. But pain doesn't have to be a life sentence.

To control chronic pain, you must deplete the pain-intensifying hormones. One way to accomplish this is through relaxation. Researchers have found that when you're in a relaxed state, pain-intensifying hormones dissipate. Try the following relaxation techniques to ease your chronic pain.

**Use your breath.** Deep breathing can derail stress, which in turn minimizes pain. Sit in a comfortable chair and place one hand on your chest and one hand on your stomach. Inhale. If the hand on your chest rises more than the hand on your stomach, you're breathing too shallowly. Breathe in deeply again, this time focusing on moving the hand on your stomach, not your chest. Practice deep breathing in this way for about two minutes three times a day.

**Master meditation.** Meditating for 5 to 10 minutes a day can help provide significant relief because it changes your perception of physical pain.

To meditate, sit in a comfortable position on the floor with your back against a wall or in a chair with your feet on the floor and your hands resting on your thighs. Breathe in slowly and deeply for five counts, then exhale slowly for five counts. Close your eyes and concentrate on a soothing, peaceful activity or place where you feel safe and calm.

**Relax to music.** Listening to music that relaxes or cheers you can help relieve pain.

**Stay active.** Exercise stimulates the release of endorphins, which raise your pain threshold and produce a sense of well-being. Aim for 20 to 30 minutes of aerobic activity six times a week. (If your pain gets worse, consult your doctor.)

## Fibromyalgia

Doctors describe fibromyalgia as a pain syndrome. What hurts are the fibrous tissues of the body: muscles, ligaments, tendons, and fasciae (sheets of connective tissue).

Fibromyalgia makes certain points on your body exquisitely sensitive to touch. These tender spots often include the inside edges of the shoulder blades, the base of the head, the outer forearms just below the elbows, and the insides of the knees.

If you have fibromyalgia, use the following strategies to help you feel better, reduce your soreness, and regain your energy.

**Take to your tub.** Heat relieves fibromyalgia pain. Draw a comfortably hot bath, then climb in for a long soak.

**Modify your breathing.** A technique called diaphragmatic breathing relaxes tight muscles and improves circulation. Allow the area below your rib cage to expand as you inhale and contract as you exhale. Continue for five minutes, doing eight breath cycles per minute.

**Stretch to soothe.** Fibromyalgia pain causes muscles to tighten. Stretching loosens stiff, sore muscles and makes you feel better.

**Think progressively.** By using a technique called progressive muscle relaxation, you can relieve some of the tightness associated with fibromyalgia. Begin by gently clenching your fists until you feel the muscles tensing. Hold for three seconds, then release. Repeat, working your muscles in the following sequence: arms, shoulders, neck, face, abdomen, lower back, buttocks, thighs, calves, and feet. Repeat twice a day

**Make time for exercise.** Even though you hurt, exercise can do you a world of good. Begin with a brisk walk for 5 minutes three times a week, then gradually work your way up to 20 minutes three times a week.

**Take a one-two punch.** In one study, people with fibromyalgia who took magnesium and malic acid (found in apples) experienced reductions in muscle pain and tenderness. Begin by taking 150 milligrams of magnesium and 600 milligrams of malic acid twice daily for one to two weeks. Then gradually increase your dosage every two to three days until you reach 300 milligrams of magnesium and 1,200 milligrams of malic acid twice daily. You can buy combination magnesium/malic acid supplements in some drugstores and health food stores.

*Note:* If you have heart or kidney problems, check with your doctor before taking magnesium supplements.

## Kidney Stones

Some say that the agony caused by kidney stones is equaled only by childbirth. Since stones are much more common among men than women, maybe they're nature's way of evening the score.

The primary symptom of a kidney stone is excruciating pain in the lower back or abdomen. You may have the urge to urinate more often and experience a burning sensation when you do go. You may notice blood in your urine. You may also feel nauseated and vomit.

Sometimes kidney stones create an obstruction in the kidney or ureter. They can also cause infections that, if left untreated, can do irreparable damage to the kidneys.

Once you've developed a kidney stone, only passing it will bring relief. Here's what you can do to flush that painful pebble out of your system and discourage future formations. (You should seek a doctor's help once you've passed the stone or if the pain is unbearable.)

**Drink lots of water.** Drink at least eight eight-ounce glasses of water every day. All that fluid dilutes the chemicals in your urine so that calcium and oxalate—the two main components of most kidney stones—can't get together.

**Get lots of citrus.** Beverages rich in citric acid, such as orange juice and lemonade, inhibit calcium stone formation. Drink 6 ounces of orange juice with each meal or 10 ounces of lemonade twice a day.

**Steer clear of stone formers.** Avoid foods that contain stone-forming oxalate, including beans, beets, peanuts, and spinach.

## Migraines

A headache is to a migraine what a bicycle is to a tank. And if you've never had one, it's hard to imagine how intensely painful a migraine can be. It's not uncommon for one to drive a woman to bed for days in a dark room. They can sometimes be so severe that they cause

---

### 10 BEST HEMORRHOID CURES

Hemorrhoids are funny, all right. Funny as a crutch. These swollen blood vessels that form in or around the anus, often in response to the physical changes triggered by pregnancy or by chronic straining to have a bowel movement, can cause excruciating pain and itching.

So when hemorrhoids act up, you need relief—fast. Below are 10 simple but speedy remedies from Martha Kershaw, M.D., assistant professor in the department of family medicine at the University of Michigan Medical Center at Ann Arbor.

1. To soothe pain and swelling, put a wet washcloth inside a plastic bag and then into the freezer until it freezes. Then take it out of the bag and apply it to the anal area for 10 minutes. "Cold makes blood vessels constrict," says Dr. Kershaw.

2. To relieve itching, apply an over-the-counter hemorrhoidal cream or ointment that contains a numbing medicine such as pramoxine 1% (like Anusol and Hemorid).

3. To reduce inflammation, apply 1% hydrocortisone cream or ointment twice a day. Use after a bowel movement or bath.

4. Soak a cloth in witch hazel and apply to the anal area for 10 minutes.

5. Sit in a bathtub of comfortably hot water for 10 to 15 minutes three times a day. Draw your knees toward your chest so that the water can reach the anal area.

6. If you have external hemorrhoids, use a cotton ball to dab them with an antifungal powder or cornstarch two or three times a day to keep them dry.

7. Avoid constipation. Drink plenty of water and eat high-fiber foods. You can also use a fiber supplement to keep stools soft and regular.

8. Switch to toilet tissue that has added moisturizers.

9. If you can stand instead of sit, do so. Sitting for long periods can aggravate hemorrhoids.

10. Learn to sleep on your side. Lying on your back places your hemorrhoids below the level of your heart. Consequently, blood flows to that area, which increases swelling.

## WOMEN ASK WHY

### *Why are migraines more common in women than in men?*

You can thank Mother Nature for that. She's the one who provides the estrogen that feeds migraines, the mother of all headaches.

Before puberty, girls and boys get migraines at about the same ratio. But once those hormones kick in, it's a different story. Then the female rate jumps to four times that of males.

The odds decrease once again as women approach menopause. When menstruation ceases and hormone levels become more steady, migraines usually occur less frequently and can even go away altogether.

A word of caution: If you have migraines and opt for hormone replacement therapy, your migraines might come back.

*Expert consulted*
*Patricia Solbach, Ph.D.*
*Director of the Center for Clinical Research*
*Menninger Clinic*
*Topeka, Kansas*

nausea, vomiting, weakness, and sensitivity to light.

For about 5 to 10 percent of women, a migraine announces its pending arrival with an aura, a visual disturbance characterized by brightly colored lines, flashes of light, dots, or spots. The pain itself can last anywhere from four hours to three days.

Once a migraine gets a foothold, it doesn't want to leave. The following measures can provide some relief and, even better, reduce the frequency and severity of recurrences.

**Take a whiff of apple.** In one study of people with migraines, the scent of green apples made their migraine pain fade. The reason why is unclear.

**Freeze the pain.** Cold helps constrict expanded blood vessels and block pain messages to your brain. Wrap ice or an ice pack in a towel and apply for 10 minutes to the area of your head that hurts.

**Consider a coffee cure.** Like ice, the caffeine in coffee constricts expanded blood vessels in the brain. But limit yourself to one five-ounce cup, which contains about 100 milligrams of caffeine. Too much coffee can aggravate a migraine.

**Mind your magnesium.** Italian researchers have found that people who get migraines tend to have lower blood levels of magnesium than people who don't. Good food sources of the mineral include green leafy vegetables, legumes, seafood, and nuts.

**Steer clear of trigger foods.** You can minimize the frequency and severity of migraines just by avoiding the foods known to cause them. The most common offenders: anything that has been aged, fermented, marinated, or pickled, such as aged cheese, red wine, and pickled herring. Also bypass any foods that contain monosodium glutamate (MSG), nitrates, or nitrites, such as canned soups and lunchmeats.

## Neck Pain

Imagine balancing a bowling ball on a pencil. Tough job, wouldn't you say? Now you have some idea what the human neck is up against, trying to support a 14-pound head.

While everyone gets neck pain from time to time, a pain in the neck doesn't have to be a pain in the neck. Here's what you can do to get rid of it.

**Go ice and easy.** Wrap ice or an ice pack in a washcloth and apply it to your neck for 15 to 20 minutes. The cold relieves stiffness and discomfort.

**Stay warm.** If your neck pain doesn't respond to cold, try heat instead. Apply a heating pad set on low or medium for up to 20 minutes.

**Take a look around.** Turn your head all the way to one side. Bring it back to center so that you're looking straight ahead. Repeat to the other side. Then look down at the floor, raise your head to center, look up at the ceiling, and lower your head to center.

**Wear sensible shoes.** High heels knock your spine out of alignment, which makes your neck jut forward. So wear flats or low-heeled shoes.

**Give your handbag the ol' heave-ho.** Slinging a heavy purse over one shoulder strains your neck as well as your back and shoulders. Instead, wear a fanny pack or backpack.

## Raynaud's Disease

Cold fingers and toes are to be expected in wintertime. But for women with Raynaud's disease, painfully frigid digits occur year-round, even when reaching into the freezer for the ice cream.

With Raynaud's, a glitch in the circulatory system causes tiny blood vessels in the fingers and toes to spasm in response to cold. With blood flow cut off, the fingers and toes become so cold that they ache. They also change color: first white, then blue, then back to red once they warm up.

Doctors sometimes recommend surgery to correct extreme cases of Raynaud's. Before you go that route, try these self-care measures to minimize your discomfort.

**Relax in a scented bath.** Sitting in a warm (not hot) bath helps increase circulation to the extremities. When Raynaud's hits, maximize the therapeutic power of the bath. Mix one teaspoon of combined essential oils such as birch, cypress, rosemary, and savory with a cup of milk and add to the bathwater. Cypress oil may help the circulatory system, savory serves as an external stimulant, and the birch and rosemary may soothe muscular pains.

**Put up your dukes.** If Raynaud's strikes you when walking from one heat zone to another, ball your hands into loose fists. Give your body a few minutes to adjust to the temperature change before releasing your fists.

**Make a beeline for E.** To improve circulation, take between 400 and 1,200 international units (IU) of vitamin E a day.

**Can caffeine.** Whether from coffee, tea, cola, or over-the-counter medication, caffeine constricts blood vessels and aggravates Raynaud's.

**Retrain your cold response.** This technique can help either your hands or feet readapt to cold, reducing a Raynaud's reaction. Fill two buckets or plastic foam coolers with 100°F water. Place one container in a cold area—on an outside patio, for example—and the other in a warm room. Wearing lightweight clothes, immerse your hands in the indoor water for 2 to 5 minutes. Wrap your hands in a towel, go outside, unwrap your hands, and immerse them in the outdoor water for 10 minutes. Go back inside and immerse your hands in the indoor water for 2 to 5 minutes. Repeat six or seven times every other day.

This procedure, called the submersion technique, trains your blood vessels to dilate rather than constrict in response to cold.

## Repetitive Strain Injury

It happens to typists, cashiers, and even grandmothers who spend their days knitting. If you do anything that involves steadily moving your hands, you are at risk for repetitive strain injury.

The most common repetitive strain injury is carpal tunnel syndrome, which makes your hand, wrist, arm, and elbow muscles feel achy and sore. The median nerve, which runs through the bony carpal tunnel in your wrist, becomes compressed by swollen tendons.

Repetitive strain injury can also affect your neck and shoulders. And it may be accompanied by other symptoms, including tingling, numbness, decreased dexterity, and fatigue.

Experts agree that for repetitive strain injury, prevention is the best medicine. That means scrutinizing your lifestyle and work style to identify and change those practices that may be putting you at risk. Start with the following strategies.

🖎 Rearrange your work areas at home and on the job to reduce repetitive reaching.

🖎 Alternate tasks whenever possible to avoid sequences of activities that use the same muscles and tendons.

🖎 Choose tools that fit your hands. Often, tools are designed for a man's larger hands.

🖎 If you sit for long periods of time, make sure that you have a chair that is properly proportioned for your body.

🖎 If your job requires moderate to heavy phone use, wear a headset.

If, despite your best efforts at prevention, you suspect that you have a repetitive strain injury, don't ignore it. Schedule an appointment with your doctor. Then try the following tips to help manage your pain.

**Give yourself a break.** If you're involved in a repetitive activity, take a break every 20 to 30 minutes. Roll your shoulders and massage your hands and fingers to stimulate circulation.

**Soothe with a scented self-massage.** Massage an herbal oil onto your skin from your elbow down to your wrist and hand. Look for a product that contains either Roman chamomile (not German chamomile) essential oil or rosemary and ginger essential oils. All of these oils have anti-inflammatory properties. They're sold in health food stores and some bath-and-beauty shops.

You can make your own massage oil by mixing 10 drops of essential oil to one ounce of carrier oil such as olive or grapeseed oil.

**Make your point.** For carpal tunnel syndrome, try this acupressure technique: Place the thumb of your right hand on the inside of your left wrist crease. (If your right wrist hurts more, then work that side first.) Place your right index finger on the back of your left wrist, opposite your right thumb. Probe for the most sensitive area, then apply firm pressure to both sides of your wrist, alternating five seconds on and five seconds off. At the same time, gently move your left hand from side to side.

To increase the pain-reducing effect, exhale or blow through your mouth when you apply pressure. Continue on-and-off applications for one minute. Repeat on your right wrist if necessary.

**Limber those digits.** To stretch the muscles and tendons in your fingers, gently press your fingertips tightly against the edge of a desk or table, bending at the base of your fingers and keeping your wrists straight. Once you feel the stretch, hold that position until you notice a change in sensation. Vary the exercise by doing it with your fingers spread apart.

**Pose against pain.** A yoga posture called the downward-facing dog creates the best skeletal alignment between the forearm and arm as well as between the shoulder and upper arm. Stand in front of a chair and put your palms flat on the front edge of the seat about shoulder-width apart. Spread your fingers so that your middle fingers are parallel and in line with your wrists. Move your feet backward until they're under your hips and your arms are straight. Bend your knees and point your tailbone toward the ceiling, creating a gentle arch in your lower back. Lower your head so that your ears are between your upper arms.

Keep your hands parallel as you slide them away from your body toward the back of the chair, straighten your knees, and balance your weight between your upper and lower body. You will feel a lengthening stretch extend from your shoulders to your wrists. Take a deep breath and hold for 15 to 30 seconds. Repeat 3 to 10 times a day. With practice, this pose will become easier and you can try turning your shoulders out and away from your neck, broadening your upper back as you stretch.

## Sciatica

Sciatica gets on your nerves in more ways than one. When you have the condition, almost every move you make is painful—standing, sitting, even hoisting a half-gallon of milk.

Most cases of sciatica result from some irritation of the sciatic nerve, which originates in the spinal cord and branches throughout both legs.

What sorts of things irritate the sciatic nerve? Often, the gel-like contents of a spinal disk leak out and press on the nerve. Arthritis in the spine may pinch the nerve. Or chemicals produced by your body in response to a lower-back injury may inflame the nerve.

Sciatica pain can last for up to a month or so. Here's what you can do help move it out.

**Create some space.** Sit on the forward part of a sturdy chair with your feet flat on the floor and your back straight. Slowly tilt your pelvis backward so that your lower back is slightly rounded; relax. Next, slowly tilt your pelvis forward so that your lower back arches; relax. Repeat four to eight times, then return to the starting position. Tilt your pelvis toward your left knee so that your weight shifts to the forward part of your left buttock; relax. Do the same toward your right knee; relax. Repeat four to eight times.

**Hit the shower.** If your sciatica is caused by a muscle strain, a muscle spasm, or another lower-back injury, try stretching in the shower. Begin by standing with your back to the spray and letting warm water run over your body for 5 to 10 minutes. Gently lean forward from your waist to the point just before pain sets in. (Hold on to a grab bar or another sturdy structure so that you don't fall.) Stay in this position for several seconds before slowly straightening up. Stand upright for a few seconds, then repeat. Finally, do the same movement to each side.

**Stretch.** Avoid sitting for long periods. Stretching movement stimulates circulation and reduces inflammation. Do this every 30 minutes.

**Get on your feet.** Walking for three to five minutes of every hour makes sciatica heal faster.

**Limit heat.** Refrain from using a heating pad or soaking in a hot bath for longer than 30 minutes. Too much heat can increase swelling and aggravate pain. Instead, opt for a cold pack wrapped in a towel every few hours for 10 to 15 minutes.

## Shoulder Pain

Women often get shoulder pain from taking on tasks that tax their shoulder muscles. When these muscles aren't used much, they stiffen and lose their flexibility. Then, when they're put to work—say, cleaning out kitchen cupboards or going for a swim—they balk big time.

Sometimes shoulder muscles become pinched between the bones and ligaments in your back, a painful condition called impingement. Then there's adhesive capsulitis, in which the shoulder stiffens so much that it can't move.

Here's what you can do to get your shoulder back in the swing of things.

**Stop what you're doing.** At the first sign of

---

### GIVE YOUR BACK A BREAK

Whether it's a heavy handbag hanging off one shoulder or a child resting on one hip, women have a habit of letting one side of their bodies carry all their burdens, says Lois Buschbacher, M.D., a physiatrist in Indianapolis.

And when you hoist a heavy purse on your shoulder, you automatically lift the weight-bearing shoulder, causing your neck muscles to cramp and spasm, leading to neck, shoulder, and back pain.

To avoid strain, carry everything—purses, boxes, bags, children—close to the center of your body. The simplest solution is to trade in your shoulder bag for a backpack purse.

**Use a backpack purse instead of a shoulder bag. It distributes the load evenly to both shoulders.**

---

shoulder pain, stop whatever you're doing. To ignore means you're asking for more.

**Ice it.** Wrap ice or an ice pack in a towel and apply it to your sore shoulder for no more than 20 minutes of each hour. The cold reduces inflammation.

**Preserve your flexibility.** Once your acute pain subsides, try this exercise sequence to re-

Dr. Buschbacher recommends two exercises—a shoulder roll and chest-and-shoulder stretch—to make neck and shoulder muscles stronger and more flexible, helping to prevent the neck and backache of "shoulder bag syndrome."

**While sitting or standing, roll your shoulders forward at the same time, then up and back, and then down to complete a circle. Repeat 10 times, then reverse direction.**

**While sitting or standing straight, draw your shoulders back together, with your elbows back and inward. Repeat 10 times.**

store your shoulder's range of motion. Begin with your arm hanging at your side. Raise it in front of you until it's over your head (or until you feel pain), then lower it. Repeat 10 times. Raise your arm out to the side, then lower it. Repeat 10 times. Tuck your upper arm against your body and bend your elbow so that your forearm is in front of you. Move your forearm toward

your stomach, then return to the starting position. Repeat 10 times. Finally, rotate your forearm to the outside, then return to the starting position. Repeat 10 times. Practice the entire sequence once or twice each day, as long as you don't feel pain.

## Tendinitis and Bursitis

With names like tennis elbow, housemaid's knees, and weaver's bottom, it sounds more like a Martha Stewart gardenwear collection than like a bunch of bruised joints.

Both tendinitis and bursitis are painful inflammations in and around the elbow, knee, hip, or any other joint put through repeated pressure and activity.

While both conditions are painful enough to sideline you, they will get better on their own. If you don't improve after three to four days, see your doctor. If you want a speedier recovery, try the following natural remedies.

**Stop it.** Some women are so stubborn that they'll just try to keep right on going through the pain. Don't. It'll only prolong the agony.

**Put the pain on ice.** Wrap ice or an ice pack in a towel and apply it to the affected area for up to 20 minutes. Repeat three or four times a day.

**Give yourself a raise.** Elevating the affected area above heart level alleviates swelling. So if your ankle hurts, slide a pillow or two underneath it, then lie down.

**Promote healing with herbs.** Ginger has potent anti-inflammatory properties. To make a tea from the dried herb, mix about one-half tea-

## FOLK REMEDY: DOES IT WORK?

### Whiskey on an Aching Tooth

Have a few whiskey sours too many, and you'll be feeling no pain. But you don't have to hit a few cocktails to feel the numbing effect of alcohol. Alcohol rubbed directly on an aching tooth will relieve the pain, at least temporarily.

It's true that alcohol affects the brain and alters your perception of pain, explains Angela Stengler, N.D., a naturopathic physician in Oceanside, California. This is because alcohol decreases the activity of nerve cells, blocking pain messages from reaching the brain.

In fact, you may remember seeing your grandmother rub some whiskey on baby brother's gums while he was teething—a remedy *not* recommended today. Even a little bit of whiskey can leave you feeling the effects. And since the impact of alcohol on the nervous system is measured by weight, giving even a smidgen of 80-proof whiskey to a tyke is not responsible parenting.

It's not a good idea for adults either. "Even a small amount of whiskey applied to an aching tooth could get someone in the habit of using alcohol to ease pain," says Dr. Stengler.

**RECOMMENDATION:** Forget It

spoon ginger with one cup boiled water, then steep for 20 minutes.

**Keep moving.** Pampering the affected area too much can leave it stiff and prone to re-injury if it's not up to the task that you set for it. So once the initial pain subsides, continuously do gentle exercises to keep the area flexible.

## Toothache

Any number of things can make a tooth hurt. But most often, the culprit is tooth decay.

A toothache should never be ignored. If you get one, call your dentist right away. The following remedies can keep you comfortable until you get proper medical attention.

**Swoosh and spit.** If the area around a tooth begins to swell, rinse your mouth with warm water. The water just might flush out debris that's irritating your gums.

**Try some cloves.** Put a drop of clove oil on your aching tooth. Clove oil acts as local anesthetic and antiseptic. You'll find clove oil in health food stores.

**Soothe with spices.** Mix ground ginger or ground red pepper (or both) in enough water to make a gooey paste. Dip a cotton ball in the paste, squeeze out any excess, then apply the cotton directly to the sore tooth. The heat generated by this remedy acts as a counterirritant to the deeper pain. Don't let the paste touch your gums, as it can be very irritating to sensitive tissue.

If this mini-compress feels too hot, rinse your mouth and discontinue use.

**Make a move.** Twenty-five minutes of aerobic activity can trigger the release of endorphins, feel-good brain chemicals that can temporarily help subdue the pain.

# Fast First-Aid

**A**ccidents happen. And for many of us, they happen in the kitchen.

Charlotte S. Yeh, M.D., rates the kitchen as one of the most hazardous rooms in the home. "Cooking, washing dishes, and even taking out the trash can lead to burns, cuts, and similar minor injuries," says Dr. Yeh, an emergency physician at the New England Medical Center in Boston. Another risky area is the bathroom. "Older women, in particular, are prone to falls in the bathroom that sometimes result in sprains," she notes.

Of course, minor medical emergencies—from cuts and scrapes to burns and bruises—occur not only at home but also on the job, on the road, and on playing fields. The best way to be prepared to handle them is to have a well-stocked first-aid kit at home and in your car. Dr. Yeh suggests that you include the following items.

- Adhesive bandages
- Antibiotic cream and/or ointment
- Chemical cold packs
- Disposable gloves
- Elastic bandages
- Gauze and adhesive tape

- List of emergency phone numbers
- Scissors with rounded tips (to cut bandages to fit)
- Triangular bandage (to make a sling)
- Tweezers

To complete your kit, add a bottle of ipecac syrup (an antidote for poisoning), a small bottle of tea tree essential oil (a natural antiseptic), a few 500-milligram capsules of ginger (to relieve motion sickness or nausea), and a bottle of homeopathic Arnica 30C (for bumps, bruises, and muscle strains), according to Connie Catellani, M.D., medical director at the Miro Center for Integrative Medicine in Evanston, Illinois. With these items handy, you will be ready to handle any minor emergency fast, if you know what to do. So read on to learn how to become an amateur at-home first-aid administrator.

## Bee Stings

Bee stings aren't always a casual mishap of summer. Some people can have life-threatening allergic reactions to bee stings. If you develop

## FOLK REMEDY: DOES IT WORK?

### Mud on a Bee Sting

Leave it to Mother Earth to take the sting out of a bad encounter with a bee. Mud has long been revered for its many unusual healing properties.

While no one knows for sure when mud was first used for stings, folklore says it was probably discovered by an early settler who stumbled to the wet ground after getting a sting on the knee. When she got up, her mud-covered knee was feeling no pain.

Why mud works on bee stings isn't completely understood. It probably has something to do with its drying effect, according to Connie Catellani, M.D., medical director at the Miro Center for Integrative Medicine in Evanston, Illinois. As the mud dries, it helps to cool the sting site, which brings pain relief. It may also draw out a stinger that has been left behind.

The next time you are stung by a bee, remove the stinger immediately if possible. Then mix some dirt in the palm of your hand with clean water until you have mud. (Soil that has a lot of clay in it works best.) The mud should be thick enough to coat the affected area, but not so thick that you can't feel it drying. Put the mud on the sting and let it dry, states Dr. Catellani. Leave it in place until it starts to crumble off, usually in one to two hours. One application is all that's necessary.

**RECOMMENDATION:** Worth a Try

with them.) For run-of-the-mill stings, here's what to do.

**Do some home surgery.** If you are stung by a honeybee, you first have to remove the stinger, the sooner the better. Using a credit card, a dull knife, or the back of your thumbnail, scrape your skin beneath the stinger until it comes out. Avoid squeezing around the fuzzy part of the stinger. That's the venom sac, and if you break it, you will release even more venom.

**Cover with a cool compress.** Soak a washcloth in cool water. Then lay it on the site of the sting to ease soreness and itching.

**Put it on ice.** To relieve swelling and pain, hold an ice cube on the sting for a few minutes, remove it for a few minutes, then repeat. Continue for no longer than 10 minutes. (You don't want to harm your skin.)

**Apply a healing paste.** Mix a paste of baking soda and water, then apply it to the site of the sting to neutralize acidity.

**Raise the area.** If the sting becomes so swollen that it aches, elevate the affected body part. Gravity will draw fluid from the area, reducing the swelling and the associated soreness.

hives that start to multiply on your body and experience any trouble breathing, intense anxiety, all-over itching or swelling, dizziness, weakness, or sweating, get to the emergency room at once. It could mean that you are going through a severe and sometimes fatal hypersensitivity reaction known as anaphylactic shock and need a shot of adrenaline immediately. (Some people who know they are allergic carry bee sting kits

## Burns

Dripping grease, hot handles, simmering liquid, even the waffle iron, can all create a red, throbbing painful burn that can last for hours.

These are known as first-degree burns and can be treated easily at home, according to Jonith Breadon, M.D., a dermatologist and co-director of dermatological surgery at the dermatology residency program at Cook County Hospital in Chicago. If a burn is blistered, you could have a second- or even third-degree burn. Get medical attention immediately.

To stop the burn of a minor mishap, do this.

**Soak it—pronto!** Hold the burned area under cool running water for at least 15 minutes. If you aren't close to a faucet, then use whatever you have handy to cool the burn—even a cold can of soda wrapped in a clean towel. Rinse the area with cool water as soon as you are able.

**Cleanse and protect.** Gently wash the affected area twice each day, using either mild soap or hydrogen peroxide. Don't use hydrogen peroxide for more than three days, however—prolonged use can actually impair wound healing. Apply an over-the-counter antibacterial ointment, then cover the area with an adhesive strip (for small burns) or a gauze dressing (for large burns).

**Go for aloe.** If you have an aloe vera plant, break off a leaf and rub the gel from inside the leaf on your burn. Or use aloe vera cream, available in drugstores and health food stores.

**Moisturize the site.** Once the burn has healed, regularly apply a thin layer of moisturizer to reduce itching and cracking and promote healing. Choose a fragrance-free lotion.

**Increase your C intake.** Vitamin C rebuilds collagen, the skin's connective tissue, and speeds healing.

## Cuts and Scrapes

When you have a break in your skin, its natural repair system leaps into action, quite liter-

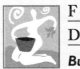

### FOLK REMEDY: DOES IT WORK?

**Butter for a Burn**

In the old days, when folks got splattered with sizzling bacon grease or touched their wrists to a fired-up barbecue grill, they dressed their burns with butter. In fact, many of us who remember our moms or grandmas using this traditional remedy are still doing it.

Stop! "Slathering a burn with butter does not reduce the pain or stop the burning," says Mary Ruth Buchness, M.D., chief of dermatology at St. Vincent's Hospital and Medical Center in New York City. "Nor does it help make it better."

Fact is, it can make it worse.

Putting butter on a burn could lead to infection, says Dr. Buchness. Because burned skin has lost its protective top layer, it is vulnerable to infection-causing bacteria. And food products—butter included—are often teeming with bacteria.

**RECOMMENDATION: Forget It**

ally. Researchers have microscopically witnessed cells moving about to fill in wounds. You can help the process along by taking steps to prevent infection and promote healing. Here's how.

**Wash away debris.** To prevent infection, hold a cut or scrape under running water until it is thoroughly clean. Don't use hydrogen peroxide for this purpose—it kills healthy skin cells that promote healing.

**Coat with a natural ointment.** Apply calendula ointment directly to the wound. Calendula has antiseptic properties. You can buy the ointment in health food stores.

**Cover up.** Covering the wound with an adhesive bandage keeps it clean and dry and speeds healing. Change the bandage twice a day.

**Slip into your second skin.** As an alternative to a bandage, try an over-the-counter product called colloidal dressing. This porous,

## FOLK REMEDY: DOES IT WORK?

### Mercurochrome for Cuts and Scrapes

Remember Mercurochrome, that rust-colored, evil-smelling antiseptic our mothers used to doctor our skinned knees? It has been replaced by medications that work.

In fact, Mercurochrome has been proven to be so ineffective that the Food and Drug Administration (FDA) has yanked it off the shelves permanently.

As its name implies, Mercurochrome contains mercury. This highly toxic substance is readily absorbed through the skin. And while the amount of Mercurochrome used to paint a skinned elbow never posed a serious health threat, direct contact with it did cause skin irritation in some people.

Mercurochrome killed less than 50 percent of the germs in cuts and scrapes—chiefly due to its alcohol content, explains Eva Vivian, Pharm.D., assistant professor of clinical pharmacy at the University of Sciences in Philadelphia. What's more, pus or blood inactivitates Mercurochrome, making it even less effective, she adds.

"You have only to stroll down the first-aid aisle of your local drugstore to find safer and more effective topical antiseptics," Dr. Vivian says. Opt for antibiotic ointments such as bacitracin and neomycin, which have been demonstrated to reduce the risk of wound infection, or products that contain FDA-approved antiseptics: alcohol, isopropyl alcohol, iodine topical solution, iodine tincture, and povidone-iodine (such as Betadine).

**RECOMMENDATION:** Forget It

lavender essential oil with one ounce of aloe vera juice (available in health food stores). Pour the solution into a spray bottle and refrigerate. Use the spray to ease pain while you heal.

## Frostbite

Most people think of frostbite as a cold-weather hazard. But the air doesn't have to be all that cold for a person to get frostbite. High winds can reduce temperatures to dangerously low levels, what we know as the windchill factor. So even if the thermometer says 20°F, a 40-mile-per-hour wind can create a windchill index of −20°F conditions. And frostbite can happen in temperatures of just 10°.

Your hands, feet, ears, nose, and other extremities are the first to feel the chill. Once your skin freezes, small icy crystals form and destroy the skin cells. This causes your blood to clot, cutting off circulation to the area. Your flesh hardens, your skin becomes waxy and white, and you lose all feeling in the affected area.

If you suspect that you have frostbite, treat it immediately by following these steps. And see your doctor as soon as possible—you can't tell how serious the damage is just by looking at your skin.

**Seek shelter.** If you notice your skin turning waxy white, get inside before frostbite develops in other areas. If you can't head indoors and you are with someone, cozy up to keep your extremities warm. Sharing body heat can help prevent

gelatin-like material sticks to your skin, creating a breathable membrane over the wound. Plus, it contains an antimicrobial medication, which fights infection. Experts say that these dressings can cut healing time in half.

**Make a soothing spray.** Mix 15 drops of

frostnip (when your skin is numb and cold but not frozen) from developing into frostbite.

**Loosen up.** As your skin thaws, it will swell. So once you are inside, remove all constrictive clothing and jewelry.

**Leave the area alone.** Rubbing frostbitten skin only does more damage. Don't even touch it.

**Don't refreeze it.** Frostbite does its harm when your skin thaws, then refreezes. So don't thaw out your skin unless you know you are staying inside.

**Stay away from fire.** Your frozen nerve endings won't be able to warn you if you start to burn your skin, so don't try to warm yourself over a flame.

**Get into warm water.** Once you are certain that you won't refreeze the affected area, gradually immerse it in a tub or saucepan of warm (102° to 105°F) water. Circulate the water to help keep it in contact with your frozen body part, and replenish the warmth continually. Warming frostbitten fingers and toes can be painful.

Once you have seen your doctor and are on the road to recovery, try these to aid healing.

➧ Rub fresh gel from an aloe vera plant on the frostbitten area. Aloe works against thromboxanes, substances that constrict blood vessels. When the vessels relax, the frostbitten area heals faster.

➧ Bandage fresh sliced beets onto the frostbitten area to ease pain and tenderness. Leave the beets on until they are dry. Repeat as necessary.

### FOLK REMEDY: DOES IT WORK?
#### Cut-and-Suck Technique for Snakebites

If a snake were to sink its fangs into your flesh, instinct would lead you to try to remove the venom one way or another. That may explain how the cut-and-suck technique, which involves making an incision over each fang mark and suctioning venom from the wound, got its start.

But it has fallen out of favor within the past 15 or so years, and doctors now believe that it does more harm than good.

"Cutting the skin may damage underlying structures such as nerves and tendons, while sucking raises the risk of infection by introducing bacteria to the wound," explains Edward J. Otten, M.D., medical director of the division of toxicology in the department of emergency medicine at the University of Cincinnati Medical Center in Ohio. "And if the person doing the sucking has any mouth lesions through which the venom can be absorbed, she is putting herself in danger as well."

Dr. Otten's advice? If you are bitten, skip the Hollywood heroics and head for a hospital emergency room instead. While some snakebite victims may have a 90-minute window before they will notice any symptoms of envenomization (the poisoning caused by a bite), many will have an immediate reaction. This can vary depending on the type of snake, the site of the bite, and the amount of venom injected. Once you are at the hospital, a doctor can determine whether you need antivenin, a medicine derived from antibodies in horses' blood that effectively neutralizes venom.

**RECOMMENDATION: Forget It**

## Insect Bites

Bugs bite because they are hungry. Like mini-vampires, they want to suck your blood.

Most insect bites are uncomfortable nuisances but not health hazards. To relieve the redness, swelling, and itching, try these natural remedies.

**Come clean.** Thoroughly wash a bite with soap and water to remove germs and allergy-provoking substances.

**Make it ice-cold.** For swelling and itching, rub an ice cube over the welt for a few minutes at a time. Repeat throughout the day as necessary. (Avoid leaving the ice in one area for more than a few minutes. It can damage your skin.)

**Take a soak.** To minimize itching, add colloidal oatmeal to a tub of lukewarm water, then climb in and soak. You can buy colloidal oatmeal in drugstores.

**Make your own repellent.** Add the following essential oils to two ounces of vegetable oil: five drops of eucalyptus, two drops of rosemary, four drops of lavender, two drops of juniper, eight drops of cedar, one drop of peppermint, one drop of clove, and one drop of cinnamon. Pour into a glass spray bottle, mix thoroughly, and apply liberally to discourage bugs from making a meal out of you. Look for essential oils in health food stores.

## Motion Sickness

Motion sickness occurs when your brain receives conflicting messages about the movement affecting your body. For example, if you are in the cabin of a boat and you can't see the choppy waves outside, everything looks still. But your inner ears and your legs sense the boat's movement. When your brain receives these conflicting messages, you feel sick.

---

### GET THE TICK OFF—CAREFULLY

You know when you have been bitten by a mosquito or stung by a bee—they leave behind itchy and throbbing reminders. But ticks don't like leaving evidence.

A tick's bite is generally painless, and a tick doesn't hit and run like other pests. Instead, a tick sticks around as long as it can, burrowing its head into your skin where it quietly feasts on your blood.

"Somewhere between 48 to 72 hours after attaching itself to your skin, the various disease-causing bacteria that a tick may carry will begin to pass into your body. So it is important to check for ticks regularly and remove them promptly," explains Ada Huang, M.D., deputy commissioner for disease control at the Westchester County Health Department in New Rochelle, New York. Some ticks carry Lyme disease and Rocky Mountain spotted fever, though it is more than likely that the tick feasting on you is not a carrier. Still, it is hard to tell, so you should get rid of a tick very carefully.

Avoid using any folk remedies rumored to coax them out or kill them, says Dr. Huang. Applying lotions or ointments might spread the bacteria. You have to keep the tick intact. Because if it ruptures, the bacteria it carries could spread. Instead, Dr. Huang suggests that you use the following technique. Use extra-fine-tip tweezers and grasp the tick as close as possible to your skin. Applying steady, firm pressure, pull the tick away from the skin. Do not squeeze or twist the tick.

After the tick is out, wash the bite with soap and water, disinfect the area with rubbing alcohol, and apply a topical

---

Probably the most annoying symptom of motion sickness is the stomach distress—the queasiness, nausea, and vomiting. Other symptoms include dizziness, faintness, fatigue, sweating, difficulty breathing, and even blackouts.

The quickest cure for motion sickness is to

first-aid antibiotic ointment. See a physician if any unusual symptoms appear. For Lyme disease, regularly examine the area for the next 30 days and if a rash appears or if you develop flulike symptoms (fever or muscle aches without a runny nose and sore throat), see a physician.

If you spend time outdoors in tick-prone areas (woods, grasses, or any place that wildlife frequents), get in the habit of checking yourself for ticks at least every night. That way, if you do find a tick, you know that it has been there less than 24 hours, explains Dr. Huang.

If you live in a state where tick-borne diseases are common, you may be interested in having removed ticks identified, particularly if you happen to remove a tick that is engorged or may have been on you for more than 48 hours. Put the tick in a resealable sandwich bag or a container and pour rubbing alcohol over it to preserve it, suggests Dr. Huang. Contact your local health department to see if your state has a tick identification service, in which case you can probably mail the tick there, and they can determine what diseases, if any, the tick may carry.

inner ears. This reduces your likelihood of getting sick.

**Control your breathing.** When you are in a situation that may bring on motion sickness, alter your breathing by inhaling for two seconds and exhaling for two seconds. This technique switches off your body's stress response, so you are less likely to become sick.

**Get to the point.** Press down on the middle of the crease of your wrist on the inside, just below your palm, with your thumb. Press fairly hard for about 10 minutes. This acupressure technique inhibits nausea and dizziness.

**Break out the band.** You can duplicate the effects of the acupressure technique described above with a modern wristband called a Sea-Band. It works by pressing a plastic stud into the middle of the underside of each wrist.

**Snap up ginger.** Ginger settles the stomach, so it can help relieve motion sickness. Take one or two capsules of powdered ginger (sold in health food stores) three times a day while you are traveling.

**Eat a little before leaving.** Consuming a light meal within two to three hours of traveling can keep motion sickness at bay.

**Choose wisely.** Where you sit in a moving vehicle can determine whether or not you get sick. Choose locations with a view of the horizon and the least amount of motion, such as the front seat of a car, the center deck of a boat, and a window seat near the wing on an airplane.

plant your feet on terra firma. Of course, that's not always possible, so here are remedies that can quiet your stomach in a jiffy.

**Keep your eyes open.** When you focus on something outside of the boat or vehicle and watch where you are going, the cues from your eyes more closely match the cues from your

## Nosebleed

For such a small body part, the nose can spill a lot of blood. That's because the blood vessels that serve your nose are very close to the surface, so they rupture with the slightest provocation.

You can almost always stop a nosebleed on your own. Here's how.

**Squeeze it dry.** Using your thumb and forefinger, squeeze your nostrils shut for 5 minutes while tilting your head forward. If bleeding resumes, squeeze your nostrils shut, this time for 15 minutes. (If you can't stop the bleeding after 15 minutes, get to a doctor.)

**Get a cold nose.** If you have been hit in the nose, wrap a bag of ice cubes in a towel, then lie down on your side and hold the ice pack to your nose.

**Get cottonmouth.** Roll a piece of tissue or a cotton ball and place it in your mouth, right under your nose, between your upper lip and gums. Leave it there for 5 to 10 minutes. The cotton applies pressure to the blood vessels that send blood to your nose.

**Forget stuffing.** Putting a wad of cotton in a bloody nose only aggravates the bleeding. The cotton attaches to the scab inside your nose. When you remove the cotton, you remove the scab, and you start to bleed again, too.

**Don't be a blowhard.** Once your nose stops bleeding, refrain from blowing your nose.

**Eat your C rations.** Vitamin C supports the manufacture of collagen and mucus, substances that maintain the moist, protective lining inside your nose. If you are prone to nosebleeds,

### IS IT BROKEN?

You slip and fall on the ice and hurt your leg. Or you tumble down the stairs and land solidly on your arm. The pain is excruciating. Your first thought: Is it broken? I have to get to a hospital or emergency center.

But wait. If you even suspect a break, the first caveat is "don't move," says Constance Nichols, M.D., emergency physician at the University of Massachusetts Medical Center in Worcester. Assess the damage first.

Bruising and swelling aren't always the best indicators of whether or not a bone is broken. A bad sprain can be very swollen, while a fracture may be only slightly swollen—at least at first. "Doctors can't always tell a sprain from a break—we often get surprised by the x-rays," says Dr. Nichols.

If the injury seems less severe, put ice on it and keep the limb elevated. If you don't get some relief within 12 to 24 hours, see your doctor.

A limb that may be broken needs to be kept still to prevent further injury.

To get to the hospital under your own steam, you will need to splint the injury to prevent further damage. You can make a homemade splint using anything that's straight and stiff, such as a closed umbrella, a golf club, short lengths of wood, cardboard, a thick magazine, several thicknesses of newspaper, or a pillow tied with a belt or rope. Follow the instructions below to secure it. Be sure to loosen the splint if swelling increases or if the area beyond the splint becomes pale or numb or throbs.

Use a pillow splint to stabilize an ankle, wrist, or hand. Position the limb in a relaxed pose on top of a pillow, and then wrap the pillow around it. Secure the splint with several strips of cloth or anything else you can tie around it to hold it in place, and then elevate.

Use a thick magazine to splint the upper arm. Roll the magazine around the arm and secure it with strips of cloth or anything else you can tie around it to hold it in place. To support the weight of the arm, make a sling by tying the ends of a long strip of cloth around the neck. The bottom of the loop should hang at about waist level so that you can easily slip the forearm through it and keep the elbow at about a 90-degree angle. For further support, splint the arm to your chest with a strip of cloth, as shown.

A heavy cardboard splint works well for a broken forearm because it keeps the arm from rotating. Fold the cardboard in thirds so that it "sandwiches" the arm, with cardboard coming up both sides. Be sure the cardboard is long enough to extend from the palm past the elbow. Place the cardboard around the injured arm, with the thumb pointing up, and secure it with strips of cloth or anything else you can tie around it to hold it in place. Once the splint is on, follow the directions above for making a sling and chest splint, which will reduce further movement.

you should take at least 60 milligrams a day (the Daily Value), which can be obtained from C-rich foods and supplements.

## Poison Ivy

It is the scourge of hikers, gardeners, and the country gentry.

If you have been exposed to poison ivy (or oak or sumac), the following tips can minimize your chances of experiencing a reaction and provide relief if you do get a rash.

**Rinse off with rubbing alcohol.** Stay outdoors and liberally splash all exposed areas of your body with rubbing alcohol. (Be careful to keep it away from your eyes.) Then wash off the alcohol with a garden hose. But act fast—you may have only a few minutes before the oil seeps into your skin.

**Disrobe in the laundry room.** As soon as you can, remove all of your clothing and thoroughly wash it in hot, soapy water. Wash your shoes, too—or at least rinse them off.

**Create a milk compress.** Soak a washcloth or a piece of gauze in cold milk, then hold it against your skin. Scientists don't yet know why this soothes a poison ivy rash.

**Dab on witch hazel.** Soak a cotton ball in witch hazel, then apply the clear lotion to the affected area of your skin.

**Discover a jewel.** The herb jewelweed reduces the inflammation associated with a poison ivy rash just as well as cortisone creams do. You can buy jewelweed cream in health food stores.

## Sprains

Doctor to patient in the emergency room: "The bad news is, it isn't broken. You have a sprain."

Many doctors say that sprains can be more complicated than broken bones. Most simple garden-variety breaks are easy to fix. You just push them back in place (sometimes surgically) until they mend together again. Sprains can be a different matter altogether.

A sprain requires two to eight weeks to heal completely, depending on how bad it is. You can assist the process by pampering the injured joint and following these tips.

**Get off it.** Putting weight on a sprained ligament can turn a partial tear into a full one. So immediately keep the injured joint up and out of harm's way.

**Just add ice.** Wrap ice in a cloth and apply it to the sprain for 20 minutes. Reapply the ice pack every few hours until the pain and swelling subside. (Avoid putting ice directly on your skin. It can cause frostbite.)

**Wrap it up.** Use an elastic bandage to compress the area around the sprained joint. This reduces swelling.

**Elevate.** Raise the injured joint above heart level to minimize pain and swelling.

**Aid with arnica.** Apply arnica cream to the sprained area as soon as possible after the injury to reduce pain, swelling, and bruising. Repeat three or four times a day for five days. This herbal cream is available in most health food stores.

*Note:* Don't use arnica on broken skin or open wounds. And don't get it in your eyes.

# PART TWO

# Look
# Your
# Best

# Win at Weight Loss

If there's one thing that women have in common, it's dieting. Talk to any woman beyond the age of 40, and chances are pretty darn good that she has been on some kind of diet at least once in her life. Our own research here at *Prevention* Health Books indicates that 71 percent of women have been on a diet in the last two years. And national surveys show that 40 percent of all women are trying to lose weight right now.

The funny thing about dieting is that, in theory, it's a pretty easy concept to grasp: Take in fewer calories than you put out, and you lose weight. Eat more than you burn, and you gain. In practice, though, we know it's an entirely different story.

One reason is that food is irresistible. For reasons too many and too complicated to go into here, women find comfort in eating and, quite often, in eating too much of the wrong thing at the wrong time.

Food is central to the good side of life. It's good food and drink (and, of course, good company) that bring festivity to celebrations, parties, family gatherings, and holidays. So it's not so

easy to take in less than you use up. Present-day lifestyles aren't helping any either.

"Women are actually exercising less," says Susan Zelitch Yanovski, M.D., director of the obesity and eating disorders program in the division of digestive diseases and nutrition at the National Institute of Diabetes and Digestive and Kidney Diseases in Bethesda, Maryland. "We sit at our jobs all day. We drive everywhere. We're eating as though we're doing a lot of physical activity, but we're not expending that kind of energy."

Not only are we physically slowing down but also our bodies' calorie-burning mechanisms, our metabolisms, are slowing as we age. After age 30, we burn 2 to 4 percent fewer calories every 10 years. Compound that with less exercise and more reasons to eat, and the scale goes up and up.

Unfortunately, there's no magic pill to melt away fat. But there is a successful formula: Healthy eating + exercise + motivation = success. "The weight comes off more gradually— about 1 percent, or one or two pounds, per week," says Dr. Yanovski. "Do it slow and easy, and it may be more likely to stay off."

It really doesn't have to be very hard. We've asked the country's top weight-loss experts for their best tips on how to eat and exercise for weight loss and where to get the motivation to follow through. We've also asked for advice on how to handle the things that derail our good intentions, like bingeing, eating out, and wilting willpower. Here's all you need to know to make it work.

## Low-Fat Living

Fat makes fat. It's as simple as that. Studies show that women who lose weight and keep it off are those who also have lost their "fat tooth."

Gram for gram, dietary fat supplies more calories than carbohydrates—nine calories per gram of fat versus four calories per gram of carbohydrates. And fat calories are more easily stored by the body than carbohydrate calories.

The rule of thumb is that you should limit your daily fat intake to 25 percent of calories. Not only does it make good weight-loss sense, it's good for your overall health as well. For a woman who consumes 1,500 calories a day, for example, no more than 375 calories should come from fat.

To get an idea of how much fat and how many calories you consume daily, take one typical day and jot down everything you eat. Then count up the calories and fat you ate using a dependable fat-and-calorie counter. Check labels on the things you're eating, too; you'll find all the numbers you need on the packages.

Based on your findings, change your eating habits according to these tips. You'll cut back on fat automatically.

**Become a part-time vegetarian.** Giving up animal foods is the single easiest way to cut

### FOLK REMEDY: DOES IT WORK?

**Slapping the Bottom of Your Chin to Get Rid of a Double Chin**

This folk remedy was likely born of a frustrated woman's ongoing war with the three villains of vanity: age, gravity, and weight gain. Whenever her chin looked like it was gaining on her, she would try to force it back into its original position with a few gentle backhands. And it even looked like it worked—for a minute or so.

Slapping the underside of your chin will cause the delicate tissues along your jaw to inflame and swell. This temporary swelling can give the illusion of firmer skin. As the swelling goes down, however, the sag reappears.

The truth is, this little exercise can do more harm than good. "Over time, the swelling can actually stretch your skin and lead to more sagging," says Debra Jaliman, M.D., clinical instructor of dermatology at Mt. Sinai Medical Center in New York City. "As women age, their skin loses its elasticity, while fat commonly collects and redistributes itself in different parts of the body. And for some, fat settles around the neck, creating a visible fold of fat beneath the jawline known as a double chin."

Even thin people are at risk for double chins if they don't have sharp angles between their jawlines and necklines, says Dr. Jaliman. Those who are genetically predisposed to having a full face, even if they maintain a nearly ideal body weight, may come face-to-face with a double chin as they age.

**RECOMMENDATION: Forget It**

fat and calories. And you don't even have to go whole hog, so to speak. Just eating one or two meatless meals per week will help.

**Give meat a supporting role.** When you do include meat in your meals, treat it as a side dish rather than as the main course. Think of your dinner plate as having three compartments, like one of those divided paper plates. Put the meat in one of the smaller compartments rather than in the big one. Fill the big one with vegetables. Put grains in the remaining compartment, allowing them to spill over into the veggies. Redesigning your plate in this way automatically slashes fat grams and calories to healthy levels.

**Halve the fat in home cooking.** You can eliminate as much as half of the fat from a recipe without altering its taste. Substitute kidney beans for half of the meat in chili. Replace half of the cheese in lasagna with spinach. Trade in sour cream for yogurt in casseroles, sauces, and dips. Use apple-sauce instead of some or all of the oil or margarine in cakes, muffins, and breads. Experiment with quantities until you're satisfied with the taste and texture.

**Add a bit of butter.** Using just one teaspoon of butter wisely can satisfy your tastebuds. For instance, add fresh crushed herbs to one teaspoon of melted butter to create a richly flavored sauce for broiled fish.

**Keep healthy foods handy.** If you work in an office, stock your desk with low-fat foods such as single-serving cans of tuna and dehydrated soups. Then on days when you don't have time to pack your lunch, you have a fast

---

### REAL-LIFE SCENARIO
#### She's on the Wrong Diet Track

Arlene has struggled with her weight since junior high school. In college, she managed to keep her weight under control by fasting for days at a time. In her twenties and thirties, she tried every celebrity diet with little success. A few years ago, she tried the prescription drug combination Fen-Phen (fenfluramine and phentermine) before it was withdrawn due to health hazards. Now, she's taking an over-the-counter herbal supplement that's supposed to help peel off the pounds safely and naturally. She's been taking the pills for a couple weeks, and they seem to work. Has Arlene finally found a natural way to control her weight?

No way. Like many women, Arlene is taking the quick-fix approach to weight loss. That she's chosen a "natural" appetite suppressant is irrelevant. Diet pills aren't a long-term solution for someone like Arlene. She may be losing weight now, but it will creep back on when she stops taking the pills.

More important, over-the-counter herbal appetite suppressants, so-called natural products, can be ineffective. The Food and Drug Administration (FDA) classifies herbal appetite suppressants as dietary supplements. Since dietary supplements aren't FDA-regulated, most "natural" diet pills haven't undergone the rigorous FDA approval process. This means that they haven't been proven to be effective.

Or safe. Some natural appetite suppressants contain ephedra (also known as ma huang). This herb contains ephedrine, an amphetamine-like substance that can raise blood pressure and speed up the heart. Since 1997, the FDA has logged more than 800 reports of side effects, from heart

---

and healthful meal right at your fingertips. You won't be as tempted to head for the nearest vending machine or fast-food outlet for a bite to eat.

**Use a fork, not your fingers.** How many cookies and potato chips can you eat with a fork? Except for raw fruits and vegetables, avoid finger palpitations to heart attack, linked to the use of ephedra. This herb has also caused at least 22 deaths. Herbal fen-phen, a "natural" version of the now-notorious diet-drug duo, is no better. It, too, contains ephedra.

Reacting to FDA warnings about ephedra's safety, many manufacturers of appetite suppressants have stopped using this herb in favor of new "natural fat burners," such as the mineral chromium picolinate and the herb garcinia. Neither has been proven to work.

Arlene should tell her doctor that she's using over-the-counter appetite suppressants, especially if she's taking other medications. Diet pills can react with many prescription drugs, including blood-pressure medications and certain antidepressants. More important, Arlene should be evaluated by her doctor for heart problems that may have occurred as a result of her taking Fen-Phen. Fenfluramine, a component of Fen-Phen, was taken off the market because it can cause heart-valve problems. Luckily, most people who took Fen-Phen or a similar drug, Redux (dexfenfluramine), short-term—for a month or two—don't seem to develop serious problems.

In order to lose weight and keep it off, Arlene has to stop using temporary solutions such as pills, fasting, and fly-by-night diet plans and change her eating and exercise habits for the long term.

**Expert consulted**
*Susan Zelitch Yanovski, M.D.*
*Director of the obesity and eating disorders*
*program*
*National Institute of Diabetes and Digestive*
*and Kidney Diseases*
*Bethesda, Maryland*

## Eating Out

Eating out used to be a luxury. These days, it's practically a necessity, making it the number one saboteur of all your best intentions. That's because you're at the mercy of a chef, possibly with a penchant for a little extra butter or cream or other "taste enhancers."

Some establishments identify certain menu items as low-fat or low-calorie. And they're now required to back up such nutrition claims, thanks to the FDA's truth-in-menu regulations. But a chef won't always stick with the recipe that was used to evaluate fat-and-calorie content. So you still don't know what you're getting.

Even nutrition experts have a hard time estimating the fat-and-calorie content of restaurant fare. In one study, a group that included dietitians underestimated the fat in five restaurant meals by an average of 49 percent.

Consider the following your own truth-in-ordering regulations.

**First, have a drink.** Of water, that is. A large glass of ice-cold water will help start filling you up, so you'll be less likely to overeat. Sip while you peruse the menu and drink generously throughout the meal.

**Make certain words off-limits.** In general, avoid any dish described in the menu as breaded, scalloped, crispy, fried, au gratin, or creamy. These foods are almost certain to be high in fat or calories.

**Make a special request.** Tell your server exactly how you want your food prepared, for example, without oil or butter. The vast majority of restaurants—94 percent, according to one

foods. They're usually loaded with fat—and because they pop in your mouth so easily, you'll likely eat more than you should.

**Find new favorites.** Don't eat foods that you don't like, even if they're low-fat and nutritious. Forcing yourself to eat something that you hate may turn you off to healthy eating.

survey—say that they will change the way they prepare a dish at a customer's request.

**Say, "On the side, please."** Always ask that a sauce or salad dressing be served on the side. That way, you control how much you eat. Dip your fork into the sauce or dressing, then stab a morsel of meat or several leaves of lettuce. You get all of the flavor but not as much fat.

**Turn down the freebies.** Many restaurants serve tortilla chips, crispy noodles, or other munchies to tide over customers until their meals arrive. Just set them aside. Or, even better, tell your server not to bring them in the first place. Bread is okay, as long as you resist the urge to slather it in butter.

**Eat half as much.** Restaurant portions are usually big enough to feed two people. Before you dig in to your entrée, set aside half of it to take home, and ask the server to put it in a doggie bag. If you want an appetizer or dessert, share it with your dining companion.

## Bingeing

Some women become so fat-conscious that they forget the positive and pleasurable aspects of eating. They eat salads for lunch and plain broiled fish for dinner day after day. This monotony can lead to mad fat cravings, which can turn into a full-blown binge.

A binge also can be emotionally driven. Spats at home or a bad day at work can turn into romancing with food. It's long been known that food is solace for negative feelings—usually anger, anxiety, or depression.

It wouldn't be so bad if it happened occasionally and then you got right back to your good intentions. But bingeing makes you feel even worse about yourself and sets up a vicious cycle. For some, binges can last for days. They just eat and eat and eat.

Here are some ways to binge-proof your body and mind.

**Eat, why don't you.** Starving yourself is a sure route to bingeing. Instead, start each day by filling your empty stomach with a breakfast of satiating protein, appetite-curbing fiber, and energy-boosting carbohydrates.

**Eat a little, a lot.** Instead of eating three squares a day, consider dividing your typical meals into mini-meals every couple of hours. It'll keep your from starving yourself between meals and, even though it seems contrary to logic, you'll end up eating less.

**Pay attention to what you're eating.** When you inhale a bagel or a sandwich in your car or at your desk, you don't really enjoy the food. So later, you're more likely to crave the flavor experience that you missed in the first place. Instead, take time to focus on what you're eating. Savor every bite.

**Plan indulgences.** Buy one serving of a favorite "forbidden" food—one that's intensely flavored and long-lasting, such as a half-ounce of rich gourmet chocolate. Let the chocolate melt on your tongue, and give it a lot of mouth play. By allowing yourself to enjoy a little of the food, you can thwart an all-out binge.

**See yourself rejecting food.** Visualize a situation that makes you vulnerable to bingeing. For example, imagine that you're going to be home alone with half a cheesecake left over from a recent party. See and smell the cheesecake. Let the craving develop. Then see yourself destroying the cheesecake or putting it in the refrigerator, out of sight. Practice this visualization technique two or three times a day to control bingeing.

**Use your "D" fences.** If you feel a binge coming on, use the five D's to try to ride it out.
1. Determine what's going on. Ask yourself, "Why is my desire to eat so high right now? Am I sad, angry, lonely, or in conflict?"

2. Delay your response by figuring out what is tempting you. Do you have trouble resisting lures like a party's festive buffet table or the smell of fresh baked goods?

3. Distract yourself for 10 minutes.

4. Distance yourself from the temptation. Either remove yourself or have someone remove the temptation from you.

5. Decide what positive steps you can take right now and in the future to strengthen your willpower.

**Match your food to your mood.** If you give in to the urge to binge, choose a low-fat food that matches how you're feeling. If you're angry, for example, reach for something crunchy such as pretzels or raw veggies. If you're feeling blue, go for smooth, creamy yogurt or pudding.

**Savor something spicy.** Hard as you may try, you just can't binge on chile peppers or hot-pepper sauce. Plus, spicy foods fill you up faster than bland or sweet foods.

**Freeze the moment.** You've given in to a binge, and you're about to feel like a failure. Don't. Just freeze the moment; that is, stop and think about why you're using food inappropriately. If you've polished off half a bag of buttered popcorn, stop and acknowledge your stuffed feeling. Then get up and toss out the rest. By tuning in to your bingeing and freezing the moment, you can stop the binge. And even if you don't stop eating, you have a chance to control how much you eat the next time.

**Go easy on yourself.** An evening of out-of-control eating doesn't mean that you should toss out your weight-loss goals. It just means that you've gotten sidetracked. Self-forgiveness is the first step in learning and moving on. Face your slip-up squarely and ask yourself what you've learned from it. Success or failure is not about how badly you fall down but about how well you pick yourself up and recover.

## Beating the Hungries

See if this sounds familiar: You've eaten dinner, and you feel as stuffed as the flounder that was once on your plate. Goodbye, hunger. You swear that you couldn't eat another bite. Then the dessert cart rolls up, and before you know it, you're ordering death-by-chocolate torte. Hello, appetite.

What's going on here is that you're confusing hunger, the gnawing urge to eat that you feel after a several-hour fast, with appetite, the desire to eat whether you're hungry or not. And it's appetite, not hunger, that gets you into trouble.

Appetite is a response to external cues, and in some people, it overreacts. It may tell you to eat because the clock says you should or because you're at the movies or because your co-worker just showed up with a box of doughnuts.

Recognizing the difference between hunger and appetite is important to your weight-loss success. If you eat only when you're hungry and stop when you're really full, too many fat grams and calories shouldn't be an issue. Granted, appetite is a mighty strong force to reckon with. Here are some tips to get it under control.

**Minimize your meals.** This was mentioned above and deserves repeating here. Divide your meals into five or six smaller meals. Without long absences of food, your appetite will be more content.

**Chew food thoroughly.** It takes about 20 minutes for the food you eat to enter your bloodstream as glucose (blood sugar) and turn off hunger. So slowly chew each morsel of food 10 to 15 times before swallowing. This allows you to truly savor your food and will help with its digestion. Besides, the effort you put into chewing every bite thoroughly will make you less inclined to overeat.

**Munch to Mozart.** Listening to music during a meal helps you to focus on what you're

## WOMEN ASK WHY

*Why do women have to face the scourge known as cellulite, while men don't seem to have a problem at all?*

Cellulite is a fancy name for the dimply fat that congregates on many a woman's thighs, buttocks, or hips. Of course, men have body fat, too. But theirs doesn't dimple because it has better structural support.

To begin with, men have thicker, more resilient skin than women. Our skin loses elasticity over time, partly because of declining estrogen levels, partly because of accumulated sun damage. What's more, the fibers that anchor skin to muscle are configured differently in men than in women. In men, the fibers crisscross to form a tight net that holds fat firmly in place. In women, the fibers run in only one direction. The combination of sagging skin and slack fibers allows fat to bulge outward, creating cellulite's trademark cottage cheese–like appearance.

Another reason men don't have a problem with cellulite is that they tend to carry their weight around their midriffs. Fat in this area is firmer and more dimple-proof than fat on the lower body, where women tend to carry their weight.

Whether you want to make cellulite less noticeable or stop it from showing up in the first place, your strategy is the same: Cut your caloric intake enough to produce a significant weight loss. That means cutting down on all calories, not just fat, and exercising regularly. Make sure that your workout includes 30 minutes of heart-pumping activity, like cycling, running, or brisk walking, at least three days a week, plus muscle-building strength training on the off days. As your fat stores shrink and your muscle tone improves, cellulite-prone areas will become tauter and smoother.

**Expert consulted**
*Maria Simonson, Ph.D.*
*Director of the health, weight, and stress clinic*
*Johns Hopkins Medical Institutions*
*Baltimore*

eating, and the rhythm will help you slow down. Choose slow, calming tunes; a fast beat may make you eat faster and "forget" what you've eaten. Your appetite may say, "More, more."

**No TV dinners.** Research shows that people who watch television while eating tend to eat significantly more than people who don't. That's because we're more intent on what we're watching than on what we're eating. And that doesn't suit a demanding appetite.

**Go easy on the fat.** Eating a high-fat meal may leave you craving even more fat, research suggests. A study found that laboratory animals that were fed meals of more than 40 percent fat continued to produce high levels of a neurochemical that induces fat cravings.

**Chat more, eat less.** Talking more and eating less is one expert's advice to prevent overindulging at mealtime. The conversation may pull your attention away from the food and add some time between each mouthful.

## Help for Trouble Zones

If you need motivation to get out and exercise, try this: You can diet all you want, but only exercise is going to trim the flabby arms, fleshy thighs, bigger bottom, and jelly belly you have acquired over the years.

Mother Nature once again can take the rap for bestowing women with these trouble zones. An enzyme called lipoprotein lipase actually directs fat to your hips, buttocks, and thighs for your body to use during pregnancy. Aging augments the problem. As you get older, your body produces less collagen and elastin, the connective tissues that enable skin to stretch and contract. Without these substances, your skin starts to sag, taking on a flabby appearance.

The good news is that you can sculpt your body's trouble zones. In addition to maintaining a healthful diet, though, you must exercise steadily and aerobically as well as do some resistance training. Here are the basics to get you started.

**Put your heart in it.** *Aerobic* describes any activity that increases your heart rate, works your heart and lungs, and burns fat. Vigorous walking, jogging, and bicycling qualify, as do dancing and gardening. Aim for at least 30 minutes of aerobic exercise three times a week.

**Add some resistance.** Resistance training tones and strengthens muscle mass, the infrastructure of your trouble zones. It also gives your metabolism a long-term boost by prompting you to build more muscles, which in turn burn more calories even when you're at rest. Experts suggest that you alternate your aerobic and resistance-training workouts. So if you walk Mondays, Wednesdays, and Fridays, do resistance training on Tuesdays and Thursdays.

**Aim for the abs.** If you have a flabby abs area, here's some good news: Abdominal fat is more metabolically active than lower-body fat, so it's easier to lose. Ordinary walking can help, but try to put in an extra effort. Add 10 to 15 more minutes to your regular walking routine. You can also try these two classic ab exercises that will help work your upper and lower abdominal muscles. To start, do one set of 8 to 15 repetitions three times a week. Gradually add more sets as you progress and work up to five times a week.

For upper abs, lie on your back with your knees bent, your feet flat on the floor, and your arms at your sides. Press your lower back onto the floor so that there is no space between your back and the floor. Slowly raise your head and shoulders from the floor and reach forward with your arms, curling your trunk as much as possible until your fingertips touch your knees. Hold for 5 to 10 seconds, and then return to the starting position. To keep your chin away from your chest while doing this exercise, imagine you are holding a small ball beneath your chin.

For lower abs, lie on your back with your knees bent and your arms crossed over your chest. Keeping your lower back flat and knees bent, raise your legs off the floor until your calves are almost parallel to the floor. Flex your feet and hold this position for 10 to 20 seconds. Make sure to breathe while holding this position. Slowly lower your legs and repeat.

## Motivation

No amount of good intentions can possibly matter if you don't have the motivation to make it through the long haul. Motivation is everything. No, it isn't always going to be easy, but we can tell you that there are (literally) tons of women out there who persevered and have been successful at losing. Here are a few tips from them on how they made it happen.

**Go by feel, not by the scale.** Do your rings feel looser? Do your pants feel less tight around the waist? Watching yourself melt back into a favorite outfit is a much bigger motivator than watching the scale. Scales, in fact, have been found to be downright discouraging.

**Take it easy.** Many women sabotage themselves by expecting too much, too fast. Try for two pounds a week, max.

**Reward your efforts.** Each time you meet a goal, no matter how small, treat yourself to something special. Pampering is always a nice reward. Get a manicure or massage.

**Don't get in a rut.** Don't do the same thing over and over. For every milestone you hit, change the way you achieved it. For example, buy a new low-fat cookbook to get some new recipes. Or walk in the community park instead of around your neighborhood. Or choose a new tape to listen to while you're pedaling your stationary bike.

**Picture yourself thin.** Visualize yourself losing weight. Imagine how you would feel and what your body would look like. This programs the subconscious mind to do what you want.

**Recruit a weight-loss buddy.** By pairing up with someone, be it a family member or friend, you become accountable to that person. So you're much less likely to blow off a workout. Choose someone who's at a similar level of fitness so that you can keep up with each other and share the satisfaction of each other's progress.

## Losing the Last Five Pounds

Pound by pound, inch by inch, you've become slimmer and more fit—until you got to the dreaded last five pounds. It's been weeks and weeks, and you're beginning to believe they're here to stay.

Don't give up. You just need an extra nudge. What's happened is that your eating and exercise habits have stayed the same, but you haven't. You're smaller now. Your body needs fewer calories to function. So the weight-loss program that took you from, say, 160 pounds to 130 may not be enough to get you to your final goal.

You have to shake things up a little. You have to burn more calories. Don't worry, it's not as hard as it sounds. Here's what to do.

**Recheck your portion size.** As you've been slimming down, it's likely that you've goosed up your eating just a tad, which didn't matter until now. Spend a few weeks eating prepackaged low-fat meals. The food label will tell you exactly what you're getting.

**Limit your snacks.** The snacks you've been enjoying may have gotten you to the weight you are now, but they could be stopping you from moving on. So forgo the low-fat cookies and crackers. Instead, get acquainted with oranges, carrots, and air-popped popcorn.

**Add some rev to your metabolism.** Come on, you can do it. Anything over 30 minutes is fat-burning time, so just go an extra 10 to 15 minutes during your workout.

**Try something new.** You're not the only one who gets bored riding a stationary bike. Your muscles do, too. If you always work the same muscles in the same way, they become very efficient and don't burn as many calories as when you first started an activity. Work your muscles in new ways by cross-training. If you've been walking, try swimming. If you've been running, try cycling. No one activity should ever become too easy.

**Change your routine.** Find little ways to increase your physical activity throughout the day. If you walk to work, for example, tack an extra block onto your route. Take the stairs instead of the elevator. And when you go to the supermarket or mall, park your car at the far end of the parking lot.

# Ageless Skin

ost of us will tolerate lines at the supermarket, the bank, and the movie theater. But lines on our faces? Get them out of here!

Well, that's a little easier said than done (though not impossible). You see, by the time tiny creases and crinkles on our skin become visible, a lot of irreversible changes have already occurred in our skin. In fact, these changes began years earlier, in our late twenties and early thirties. And they will continue as we get older and our skin gets drier, less resilient, and more fragile.

It's called aging. We can't stop it, but we can slow it down.

Of all of the things that influence the health and appearance of your skin, none is as destructive as the sun, according to Gloria Graham, M.D., a dermatologist in Morehead City, North Carolina. By one estimate, at least 80 percent of all visible skin aging results from a lifetime of repeated sun exposure.

## Ageless Ideas

"To get some idea of the effects of sun exposure, take a look at the skin on your breasts or abdomen," Dr. Graham says. "That's how your skin would look now if you had protected it."

We can't erase the damage that Old Sol has already done. But with sensible self-care, we can minimize its impact and keep our skin smooth, firm, and vibrant. Dr. Graham recommends these anti-aging tactics.

❧ Stay out of the sun, especially from 10:00 A.M. to 4:00 P.M., when the sun's rays are most intense.

❧ When you do head outdoors, wear sunscreen. Choose a product with a sun protection factor (SPF) of at least 15 and apply it at least 30 minutes before you go outside.

❧ Wear protective clothing. In general, tightly woven fabrics, like that found in a heavyweight T-shirt, screen out the sun's rays better than loosely woven fabrics.

❧ Wear sunglasses and a hat or visor.

❧ Avoid tanning beds.

❧ Keep your weight stable. Repeatedly losing and gaining causes skin to sag.

❧ Avoid cosmetics that clog the skin's hair follicles, causing blemishes. Look for products labeled "nonacnegenic" (won't provoke acne) and

## FOLK REMEDY: DOES IT WORK?

### Vinegar for Sunburn

Many a mother has poured vinegar on her kid's sunburn, hoping to provide some soothing relief. If yours was one of them, you may be wondering if the days of smelling like a pickle were worth it.

Probably not, says Jonith Breadon, M.D., a dermatologist and co-director of dermatological surgery at the dermatology residency program at Cook County Hospital in Chicago. "Pouring vinegar on a sunburn wouldn't be hurtful, but it doesn't make sense that it would be helpful either," she says. What you need is an anti-inflammatory because it is the inflammation under your skin that's causing the redness and pain. Vinegar has no anti-inflammatory qualities.

Possibly the reason moms thought it was helpful was because it felt a bit cool going on, although the sensation didn't last very long.

**RECOMMENDATION:** Forget It

---

sun. But my skin looks better, and I feel better. I've become a believer." She suggests the following nutrition prescription.

♪ 5,000 international units (IU) of vitamin A daily. A deficiency of vitamin A can leave skin rough and scaly.

♪ 500 milligrams of vitamin C daily. Vitamin C supports the formation of collagen, the connective tissue that gives skin its structure and tone.

♪ 400 IU of vitamin E daily. An antioxidant, vitamin E helps protect the skin against sun damage.

♪ 200 micrograms of selenium daily. People with low levels of selenium appear most prone to skin cancer.

## Age Spots

Don't let their name fool you: Age spots have nothing to do with age. Rather, these flat, brown patches result from overexposure to the sun.

You can easily prevent age spots just by slathering on sunscreen before heading outdoors. Unfortunately, truly protective sunscreen products didn't appear on the market until the early 1980s. So anyone born before then is likely to develop age spots.

You can take steps to fade existing spots and discourage new spots from forming. Here's what to do.

**Make 'em fade.** Apply a fade cream that contains 2 percent hydroquinone. It will help diminish age spots, although they won't disappear completely. Follow the label directions carefully.

**Discover AHAs.** To lighten age spots and to even out your skin tone, apply a cream or lotion

---

"noncomedogenic" (won't provoke blackheads and whiteheads).

♪ Remove makeup adequately and thoroughly.

♪ Use an abrasive sponge (like a loofah or Buf-Puf) to get rid of dead skin cells and open the skin's hair follicles. Keep the sponge away from the delicate area around your eyes.

♪ If you smoke, quit. Smoking depletes vitamin C from the skin, and repeatedly pursing your lips around a cigarette causes wrinkles around the mouth.

Certain nutritional supplements can also help keep your skin healthy and young-looking. "I've started taking supplements myself for my skin," Dr. Graham says. "I used to think I didn't need to because I never spent a lot of time in the that contains alpha hydroxy acids (AHAs). These natural acids strip away dead skin cells and prompt the growth of fresh, new cells. Choose a 5 percent AHA preparation and, when applying, be careful to avoid your eyelids.

**Wash your hands after handling food.** Celery, limes, and other foods contain psoralens, chemicals that can cause a sunburnlike reaction in the skin when exposed to sunlight. The affected skin eventually blisters and heals with hyperpigmentation (darker skin), which can persist for weeks to months.

**Monitor medicines.** Certain drugs make your skin more sensitive to sunlight, so you are more likely to develop age spots. Among the offenders are Retin-A, used for acne and wrinkles; antibiotics such as tetracycline; and blood pressure and diabetes medications.

## Blemishes

Much to many a woman's chagrin, blemishes don't confine themselves to teenage faces. If conditions are right, they will intrude on adult complexions, too.

Blemishes seem to come and go with hormonal fluctuations. Don't believe those stories that blemishes come from eating greasy foods or having poor hygiene. Such claims are groundless. In fact, as for hygiene, washing too often can irritate the skin and aggravate acne.

Products containing benzoyl peroxide or salicylic acid dry out blem-

### REAL-LIFE SCENARIO
#### *Take This Fair-Weather Warning*

Janet loves being outdoors—golf in the summer, weekends at the shore, and relaxing afternoons reading on her patio. And with her olive skin and dark hair and eyes, Janet doesn't bother with the heavy-duty sunscreen that her fair-skinned golfing buddy relies on to avoid getting burnt. She uses a suntan lotion with a sun protection factor (SPF) of 8 and a little moisturizer, and so far, she has never had a sunburn. How safe is Janet—really—from the sun?

Janet's right about one thing. She doesn't carry the risk of sunburn and skin cancer that her blonde buddies do, but she certainly has no room to be smug about it either. She is not immune to damage from the sun's rays.

Janet's natural coloring, the result of a skin pigment called melanin, is a barrier to the ultraviolet ray known as UVB that's associated with skin cancer. These UVB rays, which generally peak between 10:00 A.M. and 2:00 P.M., are partially absorbed by melanin, giving Janet one up on her fair-skinned friend. But the fact that African-American women can get skin cancer in spite of their darker skin proves that women of all shades need extra UVB protection. So Janet should wear a sunscreen with an SPF of 15 or higher before heading outdoors.

Here's something else Janet obviously doesn't realize. The type of ultraviolet rays that causes aging, UVA, are not blocked, even partially, by melanin. What's more, UVAs are always present, rain or shine.

If Janet wants to maintain that bronzed look year-round without the risk of wrinkles and spots, she should try a self-tanning lotion. Otherwise, there is a chance that she just might get burnt in the end.

*Expert consulted*
*Dee Anna Glaser, M.D.*
*Assistant professor of dermatology and*
*    internal medicine*
*St. Louis University School of Medicine*

ishes so that they go away faster. But benzoyl peroxide, in particular, can irritate the skin. To combat breakouts naturally, try these self-care measures.

**Put your washcloth away.** For daily care, wash your face (including underneath your chin) with a pH-balanced sensitive-skin cleanser and warm water. Use your hands rather than a washcloth to avoid aggravating inflammation. Rinse thoroughly. Repeat no more than twice a day.

**Come clean with steam.** A facial steam bath made with elder flowers, yarrow, and chamomile helps remove the dirt and pus that clog pores. Put a handful of each of the dried herbs in a large pot and cover with one to two quarts of water. Bring to a slow, gentle simmer. Remove the pot from the stove and set it where you can lean over it. Drape a towel over your head, creating a tent over the pot. Soak in the steam for up to 15 minutes.

**Yield to yarrow's benefits.** Put one ounce of dried yarrow in a quart jar. Fill the jar with boiling water, then cover and allow to steep overnight. In the morning, strain out the yarrow and store the liquid in a plastic bottle. Dampen a washcloth with the liquid and gently pat it on your face twice daily, morning and evening. Yarrow is a powerful herbal antiseptic.

**Fight zits with B$_6$.** Vitamin B$_6$ helps control breakouts, especially in women whose acne worsens during their menstrual cycles. You can safely take up to 50 milligrams a day.

## Bruises

Like a cut, a bruise involves bleeding. Only the bleeding occurs beneath the surface of the

---

### TAKE A GOOD LOOK AT YOUR BACK

No one knows how the little clumps of pigmented cells that make up moles came to be called beauty marks. Dermatologists eye moles with suspicion.

Though most moles are benign (noncancerous), some have the potential to develop into cancer, especially when they are irregular in shape and color.

While only a trained dermatologist—and sometimes a skin test—can tell them apart, it is a good idea to check yourself for certain changes in moles. That way, you can quickly identify changes that warrant attention, particularly since early treatment boosts rate of success and reduces your risk of having skin cancer spread to other parts of your body. You need to look for new moles *and* check preexisting ones for changes.

You can give your back a checkup by using a handheld mirror and a full-length mirror or by enlisting the aid of your spouse or a friend, says Jean Bolognia, M.D., director of the Pigmented Lesion Clinic at the Yale University School of Medicine.

When checking moles, think A-B-C-D.

*A (asymmetry).* Normal moles are symmetrical—if you draw a line down the middle of them, the halves will match. Melanomas have halves that don't match. The only exception are lesions that are solid black in color.

*B (border).* Normal moles have smooth, regular borders. Melanomas have blurred, irregular ones.

*C (color).* Normal moles have uniform coloring. Melanomas may have a variety of colors: red, black, brown, tan, and white.

---

skin, when an accidental encounter with something hard breaks blood vessels. Blood leaks out, producing telltale discoloration as well as swelling and soreness.

In general, the farther down a bruise is located on your body, the longer it will take to heal. A leg bruise can hang around for up to a month, primarily because leg vessels have greater blood pressure.

To get a good look at the back of your body, stand about one foot away from a full-length mirror in a well-lit room, with your back toward the mirror. First, check the backs of your thighs and lower legs. Then hold a hand-held mirror so that you catch your reflection and get a full view of the back of your body.

**D (diameter).** A normal mole is no bigger than the circumference of a pencil eraser. Most melanomas have a larger diameter.

If you notice any of these variations, make an appointment to see your doctor as soon as possible.

24 hours after the initial bump so that the bruise is fully developed. Then soak a washcloth in comfortably hot water and lay it over the bruise for 20 minutes. Repeat three times a day.

**Opt for Arnica.** A homeopathic remedy, Arnica has long been used to treat bruises, although no one knows why it works. Apply the cream, ointment, or oil once a day for two to three days. Avoid using it on broken skin since it can cause a rash.

**Rub in vitamin K.** In cream form, vitamin K helps the body break down blood at the bruise site and reabsorb it. Apply the cream as soon as possible after the bruise occurs and repeat twice a day until the bruise fades.

## Chafing

When body parts rub against each other, they create friction. Friction, in turn, scrapes away skin cells. Remove enough skin cells in this manner, and the body's immune system jumps into action. The affected skin becomes raw, red, and inflamed—all classic signs of chafing.

If chafing is severe, bacteria, fungi, and other microorganisms that normally reside on the surface of the skin can find their way under the skin. There, they can cause infection.

Fortunately, chafing never has to go that far, if you take care of the irritated skin early on. Here's how.

**Wash and dry.** If a workout leaves your skin sweaty and raw, jump in the shower and let the water run over the chafed area. Use an antibacterial soap to destroy bacteria, yeast, and fungi. Rinse thoroughly to wash away soap residues, which can aggravate chafing. Then set your

To minimize discoloration and encourage speedy healing, follow this advice.

**Use ice first.** Applying ice right after the initial bump can limit the size and severity of a bruise. Wrap the ice in a towel, elevate the bruised area, then ice the bruise for 20 minutes.

**Save heat for later.** Applying heat to a bruise dilates blood vessels in the area, so they can clear away blood cells and fluid. Wait at least blow-dryer on low and dry the chafed skin.

**Soften after your shower.** If your skin is raw but not bloody, apply moisturizer after bathing. The moisturizer will trap water on your skin, preventing further drying.

**Try tea tree oil.** Tea tree oil, an essential oil sold in health food stores, protects chafed skin from infection and speeds healing. Soak a cotton ball in water, apply a few drops of the oil to the cotton, then press the cotton against the chafed area. Repeat several times a day until your skin improves.

*Note:* If you have very sensitive skin, first test the oil by placing a drop on a clean area of arm skin. If you don't experience any irritation within 24 hours, go ahead and use the oil.

## Dry Hands

Spend any time in a super-arid environment, and you could end up with dry hands. The same is true if you frequently move your hands in and out of water, as when you are washing dishes.

Dry hands crack, burn, and itch. To make them feel and look better and to keep them from drying out in the future, follow this advice.

**Seek a superfatted soap.** Soaps that contain emollients won't irritate skin or strip away oils. Look on the package label for ingredients like lanolin, aloe, glycerin, and mineral oil.

**Seal in moisture.** Applying moisturizer to your hands immediately after washing them seals in the water that the skin has absorbed and helps prevent drying and chapping. Look for a lotion or cream that contains mineral oil or glycerin.

---

### THE RIGHT WAY TO WAX

Waxing is the best way to remove hair from your bikini line as well as from your upper lip, says Alla Zelikovsky, an aesthetician (beauty expert) at the Elizabeth Arden Red Door Salon in New York City. But we couldn't help asking: Isn't waxing messy, time-consuming, and (gulp) painful? Zelikovsky's response: Not if you do it right. Here's her step-by-step technique.

#### Bikini Area

1. Buy the wax. Any brand is fine, but Zelikovsky recommends beeswax (available in health food stores). Beeswax is lighter than the wax in those drugstore kits, she says. "The waxing goes faster, and it is not as messy or painful."

2. Heat the wax. In a double boiler, heat the wax until most, but not all, has melted. Melting all of it will make the wax thin, sticky, and hard to work with.

3. Powder up. Sprinkle a little talcum powder over the area to be waxed. It will cut the oil on your skin, which can keep wax from adhering to your skin. It will also make the hair stand up.

4. Do a temperature test. Drop a pearl-size drop of wax on your wrist or in your palm. If it is too hot, wait.

5. Apply the wax. Using the backside of a teaspoon, apply using "up" strokes, *against* the direction of hair growth. Using down strokes will make the wax difficult and painful to remove. Wax no more than a two-inch strip of hair at a time, and don't apply the wax too thickly. Finally, wax one bikini line at a time. If you wax both si-

---

**Slip on some gloves.** Wear rubber gloves with cotton liners when using household cleaning products.

## Dry Skin

Your skin naturally loses some water to the environment through evaporation. But if your skin has trouble retaining water, it will be prone to dryness.

multaneously, "your legs will stick together, it will be a big mess, and I won't be there to help," she says.

6. Soothe the skin. Slather the freshly waxed area with a lotion formulated with the herb chamomile, available in health food stores. "Chamomile calms the skin," says Zelikovsky.

7. De-wax the area. No matter what you do, wax will cling to your skin, says Zelikovsky. Start to remove the wax after it has hardened slightly but while it is still a little supple. Slather the area with an oily cold cream and pull off as much as you can in the direction it was applied (against the growth).

8. Wait for regrowth. Never shave your bikini line between waxings—no matter how frantic your schedule. "Shaving makes the hair like wire," says Zelikovsky.

### Upper Lip Area

1. Follow steps 1 through 4 above.

2. Apply the wax. Don't apply wax in one long line above your lip, says Zelikovsky. Rather, apply it in five separate "pieces," waxing from the corners of your mouth, in. Wax the left side of your mouth, then the right. Next, wax the left middle part of the lip line, then the right. Last, wax the area directly under your nose. To remove, pull the wax up, not down. Removing that last piece of wax can bring tears to your eyes. To make it less painful, form an extra ball of warm wax, press it to the waxed area, and pull.

3. Soothe the skin. To minimize redness and swelling, wipe the area with an antiseptic and pat with ice.

Dry, chapped, cracking skin won't protect you from viruses and infections as well as it should. So keeping it hydrated is essential. It is also quite easy to do, as these tips demonstrate.

**Moisturize with milk.** Pour cold milk into a bowl or basin, then dip a washcloth or a piece of gauze in the milk and hold it against the affected skin for five minutes. Milk soothes dry skin and has anti-inflammatory properties to relieve itching.

**Moisturize with mineral oil.** Plain old mineral oil traps moisture in the skin, helping it stay hydrated.

**Rehydrate at bedtime.** Before going to bed, soak in a lukewarm bath almost to the point where your fingertips shrivel like prunes—your skin will be fully hydrated. Get out of the tub, pat yourself semi-dry, and apply a thick layer of shortening to the affected skin. Slip into an old pair of pajamas and climb into bed.

**Cleanse gently.** For your daily shower or bath, use lukewarm water and a very mild soap. If your skin is extremely dry, avoid strong antibacterial soaps, which tend to dry skin.

## Ingrown Hair

If you shave your legs too close, you can nick the top of a hair follicle, causing it to become partially obstructed. The hair inside then grows at an angle, eventually piercing the side of the follicle and burying itself in your skin. The skin becomes inflamed and produces a tiny red bump, the familiar mark of an ingrown hair.

One can also occur when an individual hair grows straight out of its follicle, then curls down and reenters the follicle.

Whatever the cause, an ingrown hair usually heals on its own within two weeks. To speed healing and prevent a recurrence, follow this advice.

**Soothe with soap.** Wash the area around the ingrown hair twice each day with an antibacterial soap. Follow up with a dab of a benzoyl peroxide cream, found at your local drugstore. This will help reduce the inflammation.

**Change blades regularly.** If an ingrown

hair has become infected, change your razor blade each time you shave until the hair heals. Otherwise, it could become reinfected.

**Shield your skin.** When shaving, protect hair follicles from nicks by creating a moisture barrier between your skin and the blade. A mild soap will do the job, although you can also use a shaving foam or gel.

## Oily Skin

Everyone's skin has a coating of oil, or sebum, to keep out dirt and make skin soft and supple. Sometimes the oil becomes too thick, thanks to overproductive sebaceous glands.

Like dry skin, oily skin becomes a problem only when it isn't properly cared for. You can minimize the sheen and reduce the likelihood of breakouts by following this advice.

**Buy the right bar.** To wash your face, use a soap made with glycerin, cucumber, witch hazel, or citrus acids. These natural ingredients keep oily skin healthy.

**Lather up less.** Washing your face too often may stimulate your skin to produce *more* oil. Limit yourself to three times a day, tops.

**Try a natural toner.** After washing your face, apply witch hazel, using a cotton ball. Witch hazel will clean soap residues and reduce the amount of oil on your skin.

**Fight oil with (essential) oil.** Add two drops of lemongrass essential oil to one-half ounce of a carrier oil such as apricot kernel, flaxseed, or hazelnut (available in most health food stores). With a cotton ball or with your clean fingers, gently apply the mixture to your face after every cleansing. Lemongrass helps de-

### WOMAN TO WOMAN
#### She Controls Her Psoriasis Naturally

*For the past 10 years, Karin C. Holstein, 41, a former cover girl turned writer and public relations and image consultant in Miami, has used a healthy diet, supplements, and other natural remedies to control her psoriasis. Here's her story.*

I grew up in Germany and at the age of eight was diagnosed with psoriasis—a condition that causes scales and patches on the skin. At first I was lucky; my psoriasis wasn't severe. But it did get worse in my teens.

As a student in Paris, I was offered a modeling job. I couldn't believe it—a model with psoriasis? But I signed up. One assignment led to another, and I became a full-time model in 1973. I continued to hide my psoriasis, which was by this time limited to my hands, elbows, knees, and ankles.

Ironically, knowing that I could make it as a model, with or without psoriasis, was a turning point for me.

I became a vegetarian. I also began to explore natural ways to treat my condition, such as internal cleansing, exercise, and supplements. But my skin didn't clear up overnight. It took six to nine months to see results.

Now, I'm what you might call a part-time vegetarian. I eat

grease the skin and regulates overactive sebaceous glands, but keep it away from your eyes.

## Rashes

Think of a rash as your body's built-in distress signal. That red, itchy patch of skin may be telling you that you have come into contact with an irritant such as harsh detergent, poison ivy, or even rubber. Or that you are having an allergic reaction to a food or a medication. Or it may be a sign of illness.

Depending on its cause, a rash may take a week or longer to heal. You can minimize itching and discomfort, in the meantime, with fish or chicken two or three times a week, along with whole grains and fresh fruits and vegetables. I avoid processed and fried foods.

I believe that psoriasis is partly linked to a buildup of toxins in the body. Having learned in health spas about the beneficial effects of internal cleansing, I used to fast one day a week. I don't fast at all now. I do internal cleansing by drinking lots of water and by sitting in a steam room or sauna—both help eliminate toxins through the pores.

I also exercise three or four times a week. I learned that exercise triggers the release of endorphins, brain chemicals that promote a feeling of well-being. In my mind, having a positive attitude is important to overall health.

I also take vitamin and mineral supplements that keep the immune system healthy. These include zinc and antioxidants such as vitamins C and E, beta-carotene, and selenium. I also take vitamins $B_1$, $B_2$, $B_3$, $B_6$, and $B_{12}$ to help the nervous system. Cysteine, an essential amino acid containing sulfur, which detoxifies the system, rounds out my supplement regimen.

I still have psoriasis, though very little. Using natural treatments has done a lot of good. The improvement has been incredible.

these self-care measures. (If your rash gets worse after a day or two, or if it is accompanied by fever, headache, joint pain, or difficulty breathing, see your doctor right away.)

**Sit in soda.** Pour one-half cup of baking soda into a tub full of lukewarm water, then climb in for a 15-minute soak. You could also make a paste from a spoonful of baking soda mixed with a little water and dab that on your rash to soothe your skin. Baking soda helps relieve itching.

**Make a milk compress.** Combine one part milk and one part water, then soak a washcloth in the mixture and lay it over the rash. Milk's anti-inflammatory properties reduce itching. Remember to rinse off afterward.

**Consider coal tar.** Look in your drugstore for oils and gels made with coal tar, a potent anti-itch ingredient. Rub the oil or gel onto the affected skin, following the label directions. Because coal tar can stain, your best bet is to apply it at bedtime, then slip into old pajamas and sleep on old sheets.

**Cool with cornstarch.** Ordinary cornstarch can be quite soothing on a rash. Just sprinkle some on the affected skin.

## Scarring

For women who have one, a scar usually serves as a visible reminder of something they'd just as soon forget—a too-close encounter with a paring knife, a fall off a bicycle, a chance step onto a piece of glass. Injuries like these can damage the deepest layer of skin, called the dermis. When that happens, the body produces new tissue to repair the wound, and a scar forms. Scarring can also follow a serious case of adolescent acne or a surgical incision.

Whether you want to prevent scarring or fade an existing scar, these measures can help.

**Take supplemental C.** While your skin is on the mend, take 250 milligrams of vitamin C twice each day—once in the morning, once in the evening. Vitamin C speeds wound healing.

**Massage the skin.** Once the skin has healed, firmly massage the area once or twice a day for two months. Putting pressure on the injury supports the wound-healing process, making the scar less prominent.

**Butter it up.** For an existing scar, apply cocoa butter lotion or cream every day. The cocoa butter keeps the scar from becoming more prominent.

## Sensitive Skin

If you have sensitive skin, certain substances can make your skin itch, burn, sting, or break out into a red, swollen rash or tiny blisters. Among the common culprits are ingredients in skin-care products, cosmetics, and household cleaners.

Sometimes what looks like a run-of-the-mill skin irritation is actually an allergic reaction. You can find out whether you have an allergy by asking your dermatologist to do a skin-patch test.

Whatever the cause of your sensitive skin, you can reduce your chances of a flare-up by following this skin-care routine.

**Cut your bath time.** Keep your baths or showers short. Use cool or lukewarm water and a mild, fragrance- and preservative-free cleanser. Be sure to thoroughly rinse your skin to remove any cleanser residues, then pat dry.

**Stick with hypoallergenic products.** Hypoallergenic products contain fewer skin-irritating fragrances and preservatives than "regular" products.

**Leave scents alone.** Fragrance is among the most common skin irritants. Products labeled "unscented" or "fragrance-free" may actually contain fragrance to mask the odors of other ingredients. So read labels and steer clear of products that use words such as *fragrance, perfume,* or *aromatherapy* or that contain any of the botanicals, including chamomile, rosewood, lavender, lemon, and rosemary.

**Check for formaldehyde.** Formaldehyde, another common skin irritant, is found in shampoos, makeup, and many skin-care products. But you probably won't see it listed as an ingredient. Instead, read labels for quaternium #15, DMDM hydantoin, imidazolidinyl urea, diazolidinyl urea, or Bronopol—chemical additives that release formaldehyde over time.

## Spider Veins

At least 40 percent of women develop spider veins—networks of tiny red, blue, or purple blood vessels that appear on the upper thighs, behind the knees, and on the feet. They can be caused by a superficial injury, such as being hit by a tennis ball or being jumped on by a pet. They are also quite common during pregnancy: Nearly two-thirds of moms-to-be get them.

Spider veins may be unsightly, but they seldom cause the pain and swelling associated with varicose veins. You can have them removed by laser or injection. If you prefer to go the natural route, doctors suggest these strategies.

**Have a bowl of berries.** Fruits like blueberries, blackberries, cherries, and raspberries supply bioflavonoids, natural compounds that help strengthen blood vessels. The darker the fruit, the more bioflavonoids it contains.

**Don't peel away the pith.** Pith, the white membrane in citrus fruits such as oranges and grapefruit, provides a healthy dose of bioflavonoids as well.

**Go for ginkgo.** The herb ginkgo helps strengthen the tissues that form vein walls. Look for a 50:1 extract, which will be specified on the label. Take 40 milligrams three times a day until spider veins are diminished.

## Stretch Marks

Most women associate stretch marks with pregnancy. But the scarlike lesions can result from weight gain, exercises that bulk up the muscles—anything that makes the skin's elastic tissue stretch and tear. They have also been linked to prolonged use of high-potency cortisone creams and other corticosteroid medications, which cause the skin to become thin.

For stretch marks, prevention is the best medicine. Because once you have them, all the cocoa butter, olive oil, and vitamin E gel in the world won't make them disappear. The best you can do is to minimize their appearance. Here's how.

**Do the right moves.** The following exercises can firm the areas with stretch marks, making the lesions less visible. To start, do 8 to 10 repetitions of each exercise three times a week. Gradually work your way up to 20 reps three times a week.

To firm the hips and legs, lie on the floor on your side with your thighs together, top leg straight and bottom leg bent at the knee. Extend the arm that's closest to the floor over your head and rest your head on your arm. Put your other hand flat on the floor in front of your waist. Keeping your top leg straight and your toes pointed straight ahead, slowly raise your top leg from hip to toe about one foot off the ground, then slowly lower it back to the floor. Don't just jerk your leg up in the air and let it fall back down. Instead, raise and lower your leg in a slow, controlled motion. Do all of your repetitions before switching legs.

To firm your inner thighs, lie on your side, supporting your head with your hand. Keep your bottom leg straight. Bending the top leg, place your foot in front of your bottom leg. Try to raise the bottom leg about six inches, then lower it. Do all of your repetitions before switching legs.

To firm your bottom, lie facedown on the floor with a pillow under your hips. Turn your head to one side and rest your cheek on clasped hands. Raise one leg off the floor, heel first, three to six inches, then lower it. Repeat with your other leg, then continue alternating legs.

**Moms-to-be, moisturize.** If you are pregnant, apply moisturizer to your abdomen twice a day. Your skin's elastic tissue stretches more and tears less when it is moisturized, so stretch marks are less likely to form.

## Sunburn

Anyone can get sunburn, but some women are more susceptible than others. Fair-skinned blondes and redheads, for example, tend to burn easier than dark-skinned brunettes. Likewise, women taking certain medications, including birth control pills and estrogen replacement pills, can become more sensitive to the sun.

If you find yourself nursing a sunburn, the following tips can help relieve the redness and discomfort. (Be sure to see your doctor if you experience severe pain, blistering, or excessive swelling.)

**Soak in oatmeal.** To relieve the itchiness of dried, sunburned skin, add one cup of colloidal oatmeal (sold in drugstores) to a tub full of cool water. Then soak for 15 minutes.

**Apply an aloe/lavender combination.** Squeeze the gel from a whole aloe leaf and add one or two drops of lavender essential oil. Lightly apply the gel to sunburned skin. Repeat two or three times a day until the pain subsides.

This powerful antiseptic and antibacterial formula that can speed the healing process.

**Relieve pain with plantain.** An herbal wash made from plantain leaves may take away the sting of sunburn. You can buy the dried leaves in some health food stores. Grind up a few leaves, place the mulch in a cup of boiling water, and steep for a few minutes. When the liquid cools, pour or splash it onto the sunburned skin. You can use the wash once or twice a day. Do not confuse the plant plantain with the banana-like fruit of the same name.

**Ease the pain with E.** Take 400 IU of vitamin E every four hours (while awake) for one day, starting immediately after getting a sunburn. The d-alpha-tocopherol form of the vitamin works best. Studies have shown vitamin E (d-alpha-tocopherol) contains an amino acid that reduces skin damage caused by sunburn.

## Varicose Veins

Veins become varicose, or swollen, when the valves lining the vein walls fail to do their job. Normally, these valves prevent blood from flowing backward when it is making a return trip to the heart. A valve opens, the blood goes through, and the valve closes. But if that valve malfunctions, it allows the blood to reverse direction and pool in the vein. Eventually, the pressure created by the pooled blood stretches the vein wall. That's when the vein becomes visible on the surface of the skin.

Why do some women get varicose veins while others don't? It's genetics, mostly. If your mother (or father) has varicose veins, you are likely to have them, too. Your risk increases if you are overweight or you stand for six or more hours a day.

Pregnancy can also contribute to the development of varicose veins, for a couple of reasons. First, the hormonal changes that occur during pregnancy allow the veins to stretch to accommodate extra blood flow. Second, the weight of the fetus can interfere with blood flow and put greater pressure on the leg veins, especially during the third trimester.

Fortunately, you don't have to put up with unsightly veins that make your legs feel tired and heavy. These strategies can minimize your discomfort and keep varicose veins from worsening.

**Comfort with a compress.** Put one-half to one cup of distilled witch hazel in a bowl and refrigerate it for at least one hour. Then add six drops of cypress essential oil, one drop of lemon essential oil, and one drop of bergamot essential oil. Soak a cloth in the witch hazel solution, then lay the cloth over the varicose vein for 15 minutes. While applying the compress, elevate your feet on a few pillows to support circulation. Both the witch hazel and the essential oils have an astringent effect—they shrink small blood vessels near the surface of the skin, temporarily reducing swelling.

**Try aescin.** In one study, taking 50 milligrams of aescin (the extract from the dried seeds of the horse chestnut plant) twice a day for 12 weeks reduced the lower-leg swelling associated with varicose veins by 25 percent. Aescin is available at health food stores.

**Get your fill of roughage.** Every day, eat at least 25 grams (the Daily Value) of fiber. A fiber-rich diet featuring whole grains, fruits, and vegetables helps prevent constipation by making stool easier to pass. If you must strain to move your bowels, you create pressure in your abdomen that can block the flow of blood to your legs. Over time, the increased pressure may weaken the walls of the veins in your legs.

**Stock up on C.** Your body uses vitamin C to build collagen and elastin, connective tissues that help strengthen vein walls. Take 500 milligrams twice a day.

**Move your legs.** Even while you are sitting, you can do exercises to keep the blood in your legs circulating. Here's one to try: Flex your feet, lifting your toes while keeping your heels down, as though you are pumping a piano pedal. Continue for a minute or two, then repeat every hour.

## Wrinkles

We have already said it, but it's worth saying again: Unprotected sun exposure is the leading cause of wrinkles. It wreaks havoc on the skin by breaking down collagen and elastin, two connective tissues that give skin its structure and tone.

Fortunately, skin—like the rest of the body—has the capacity to repair itself. You can take steps to diminish existing wrinkles and discourage new ones from appearing. Here's what dermatologists recommend.

**Say yes to AHAs.** Alpha hydroxy acids (AHAs) fight wrinkles in two ways. First, they loosen and remove old, wrinkled cells to uncover the young, fresh cells underneath. Second, they plump the skin's surface, in essence filling in the "dents" that you see as wrinkles. Use an 8 percent AHA preparation on your face and neck twice a day—once in the morning and once at night. For the sensitive area around the eyes, use a fragrance-free 5 percent AHA eye cream and avoid getting it into your eyes or on your eyelashes. If you do, thoroughly rinse the affected eye with cold water.

**Moisturize in the morning.** Plumping the skin with moisturizer can help hide wrinkles. But most women apply moisturizer before bed, so their appearance is improved for only four to six hours while they sleep. You are better off moisturizing first thing in the morning.

**Smooth on topical vitamin C.** Unlike AHAs, which reverse skin damage by speeding up the exfoliation process, vitamin C might help prevent damage in the first place. As an antioxidant, vitamin C protects against wrinkles by fighting off free radicals, unstable molecules that form when the skin is exposed to sunlight and ultraviolet radiation and that harm healthy cells and contribute to skin damage.

Applying vitamin C directly to the skin can help prevent depletion of the nutrient when you spend a lot of time in the sun. One topical vitamin C product is Cellex-C. It's a 10 percent vitamin C solution that's available without a prescription from dermatologists and licensed aestheticians.

# Great Hair Secrets

Of all the features that make up the human body, only hair holds the honor of being celebrated in a Broadway musical. Not bad for what amounts to a mass of hard, dead protein.

The way you wear your hair helps define you as a person. There is nothing about your looks that can so dramatically change your image.

Which is why so many of us fret so over our hair. We perm it, straighten it, tease it, roll it, iron it, primp it, color it, and frizz it. Bad hair day? Yes, we've all been there.

Maybe it's time to relax a little. There is a limit to what we can do with our hair because the course of our hair—the type, texture, and color—was genetically determined at conception by Mom and Dad, notes Patricia Farris, M.D., clinical assistant professor of dermatology at Tulane University School of Medicine in New Orleans.

"Unfortunately, most women don't realize the damage that overprocessing can do to their hair," says Dr. Farris. "Even blow-drying or using any heated styling appliance makes hair dry, brittle, and prone to breakage over time."

The effects of overprocessing are compounded by the fact that hair naturally dries out with age. "As you get older, your skin's sebaceous glands don't function as efficiently," Dr. Farris explains. "Without the sebum produced by these glands to provide lubrication, your scalp and hair become drier." Your hair may become thinner, too, especially after menopause.

Even if your hair has endured years of harsh treatments, you can take steps to repair any existing damage and restore life and luster. Here's what you can do to make your hair look its natural best.

## Bad Hair Days

Okay, we'll allow that your hair seems to get a mind of its own. Curls lose their bounce. Bangs head in new directions. Nothing you do can persuade those strands to go where you want them to and stay there.

For those days when you can't get your hair headed in the right direction, here's what to do.

**Go wrong.** Wet your comb and run it through your hair in the direction opposite your usual style. Repeat a few times, then retrain your hair to go in the right direction.

**Be mist-ifying.** Fill a misting bottle (like the ones used to spray plants) with clean water. Then mist your hair, put some gel on it, and run a comb through it. No matter what gel you choose, start with less than the amount that the label instructions suggest.

**Give curls a boost.** Use a curling iron to restore bounce and body to curly or wavy hair. To prevent split ends, first cool the iron by rolling it in a wet towel. If your hair still goes limp, try boosting the curl with a little spray.

**Subdue static.** For flyaway hair, spray on a thermal styling conditioner right after shampooing and conditioning. Blow-dry your hair using the lowest setting and holding the dryer six to eight inches from your head. Or, set your hair with Velcro rollers, then blow-dry.

## Dandruff

Human skin is constantly recreating itself. The cells migrate to the surface, then slough off. Usually, this process takes about 21 days. Sometimes, though, the cells turn around in half the time (usually on the day you pick to wear your navy blue jacket) and end up forming clumps on your scalp. In no time, you're Snow White.

Here's what you can do to dwarf the problem.

**Lather your locks daily.** Shampooing cleans dead skin cells from your scalp. So the more you do it, the better you'll control your dandruff.

**Use the right shampoo.** Choose a dandruff shampoo made with tar, selenium, or zinc

---

### FOLK REMEDY: DOES IT WORK?

**Beer for Shiny Hair**

Teenage girls were rinsing their hair with beer to make it shine back in the fifties. And who knows where they got the idea? Maybe a chemistry teacher. There seems to be something to it.

One of the main reasons why your hair loses its shine is because of damage to the outer layer of the hair shaft called the cuticle. The cuticle is lined with scales that resemble shingles on a rooftop. When the scales lie smooth on the shaft, they reflect light. Because of sun exposure, overbrushing, and chemical assaults on your hair, the shingles become loose and curl upward, making hair look dull.

The protein found in beer can fill in the irregular surface between the scales of the cuticle, causing a smoother appearance and more shine, says Leslie Baumann, M.D., director and assistant professor of cosmetic dermatology at the University of Miami. For the best results, soak your hair thoroughly with the beer, then rinse. Be sure to use beer that's fresh and still foaming because the proteins necessary to make the head on the beer are the same ones that add shine to hair. Stale beer has no head because these proteins have already been broken down. And just as with any conditioner, beer's shining effect only lasts until the next washing.

**Recommendation:** Worth a Try

---

pyrithione. These ingredients remove scaly patches from your scalp and relieve itching.

**Double up.** When washing your hair with a dandruff shampoo, lather once and rinse well. Lather again, this time really rubbing your scalp. Then let the shampoo sit for at least five minutes to give the active ingredient a chance to work. Rinse thoroughly.

**Pull a switcheroo.** Use your dandruff shampoo every day for two weeks. Then cut back to every other day, alternating it with a gentle nonmedicated shampoo. This protects your hair against the drying effects of the chemicals in dandruff shampoo. (If you don't notice any improvement in the first two weeks of using a dandruff shampoo, you may have a condition other than dandruff. See your doctor.)

**Skip the conditioner.** Heavy after-shampoo conditioners make dandruff worse. So if your hair becomes dry from using a non-tar-based dandruff shampoo, alternate it with a tar-based shampoo. Tar leaves hair soft and tangle-free.

**Put moisture back.** Drinking at least eight eight-ounce glasses of water a day moisturizes your scalp from the inside out. Fruits and vegetables also help you stay hydrated.

## Dry Hair

In healthy hair, the cells that make up each strand's outer layer, called the cuticle, overlap like shingles on a roof. If the cells are roughed up or chipped away, the strand loses moisture and doesn't reflect light as it should. So hair not only feels dry but looks dry, too.

With a few simple changes in your hair-care routine, you can repair the damage that leads to dry hair.

**Be picky about shampoo.** Look for a shampoo that contains aloe, glycerin, honey, amino acids, or natural oils. All of these substances moisturize hair. Steer clear of products that combine shampoo and conditioner; they neither clean nor condition well.

**Get into condition.** After shampooing, apply an instant conditioner that has been for-

---

### REAL-LIFE SCENARIO
#### All Her Care Is Damaging Her Hair

Susan started coloring her mousy brown hair in her twenties. Now that she's 47, she uses coloring rinses even more frequently to cover up the sprays of gray that are starting to appear. Lately, Susan's hair is dry and breaks easily. She uses a shampoo with built-in conditioners, brushes 100 strokes every night with a natural-bristle brush, and conditions her hair weekly with olive oil. She also uses a spray-on "luminator" that promised to give her hair brilliant shine. But still her hair is dull and splits easily. She tries not to use her blow-dryer and curling iron every day, but without them, her hair looks even worse. Susan's hairdresser says that her best bet is to get her hair cut short and start over, but Susan likes her hair long. Short of getting a buzz cut, what more can Susan do to solve her problem?

After years of abuse, Susan's hair is sending out a desperate SOS. And it's not just 20 years of dyeing that has caused the problem. The brushing, spraying, blow-drying, and curling have all contributed. Her hair has lost its bounce and shine because the hair shafts have broken down.

But Susan doesn't have to forfeit her long locks to get her hair back in shape. Nor does she have to quit coloring it. In fact, she can replenish her hair naturally and on her own.

First, Susan should select shampoos and conditioners that contain keratin, collagen, or PVP—listed near the top of ingredients. Seaweed, also called algae extract, is also good.

For a totally natural conditioner, she can try raw egg (whipped till the yolk is blended with the white of the egg) or mayonnaise. Once a week, Susan can massage either one egg or two tablespoons of mayonnaise into her freshly washed hair, wrap her head in a towel for 10 minutes, then

---

mulated for dry hair. Such a product protects against damage from drying and styling.

**Moisturize with essential oils.** If you can't find a commercial conditioner that you like, make your own instead. Add six drops each of lavender, bay, and sandalwood essential oils (available in health food stores) to six ounces of rinse first with warm, then cool water. If Susan uses the mayo, she should add a dash of vanilla so that she won't smell like a tuna sandwich later.

Susan should also bag her hot-oil treatments. They're a complete waste of time. The molecules that make up olive oil are too large to penetrate the hair shaft, so the oil just sits on top of the hair. Same for the sprays and pomades. After a while, all that wax and silicone coat the cuticle of the hair shaft, making hair look dull and feel gummy.

To strip away this waxy buildup, Susan should do a clarifying rinse once a month. White vinegar will do the job. She should simply pour it into a spray bottle and spritz it on her freshly washed hair. After 10 minutes, she can rinse with cold water or do a light shampoo.

Finally, Susan should cut back on her 100 strokes nightly. Just a 25- to 50-stroke routine every evening is all that's needed to help the scalp get stimulated. This kind of contact also helps rid the hair of particles that it may have picked up during the day. She should continue to use her natural-bristle brush to avoid the split ends that she may otherwise get from excessive brushing. If Susan uses a metal brush while blow-drying to set her style, she should use caution. The metal absorbs the blow-dryer's heat and can singe the hair.

So when will Susan see results? Every head of hair is different, but generally speaking, she should see some significant difference after the first treatment.

*Expert consulted*
*Christopher Mackin*
*Resident trichologist (specialist for hair and scalp)*
*Elizabeth Arden Red Door Salon*
*New York City*

warm sesame or soy oil. Part your hair into one-inch sections and apply the oil blend to your scalp with a wad of cotton. Wrap your head in a towel and wait 15 minutes. Then uncover your hair and shampoo twice.

**Dry wisely.** Whenever possible, use only a towel to pat or gently squeeze water from your hair. If you must use a blow-dryer, apply a thermal styling conditioner to protect your hair. Set the dryer on high to remove residual water, then switch to low for styling. Hold the dryer at least six to eight inches from your hair at all times.

**Outsmart the sun.** To prevent sun damage, mist your hair with a styling product that contains sunscreen or a sun filter such as octyl-dimethyl PABA. And wear a lightweight, tightly woven hat with a wide brim.

**Do a pre-swim prep.** Before swimming in a chlorinated pool, apply an instant conditioner to your hair and slip on a swim cap. Afterward, thoroughly rinse your hair, then wash it as usual.

## Frizzies

If the frizzies have rendered your mane unmanageable, you can bring them under control. The key is to get your hair in top condition. Start with these strategies.

**Massage, don't scrub.** Choose a shampoo formulated for dry or damaged hair. Massage it onto your scalp with your fingertips, then gently work it through your hair with your fingers. Leave your hair hanging down as you wash it rather than bunching it on top of your head, which causes breakage.

**Gently detangle.** After shampooing, work a quarter-size dollop of detangling conditioner through your hair. (Avoid products that are heavy, waxy, or silicone-based.) Gently run a wide-toothed comb through your hair, proceeding in small sections from the ends toward your scalp. Stop when you're about an inch from

**Why does gray hair look distinguished on men but not on women?**

The easy answer: The old double standard. But according to evolutionary theorists, the true answer is more complex. It has its roots, so to speak, in sexual selection—the ways in which our Stone Age ancestors chose their mates.

Our male ancestors chose mates whose physical appearance suggested that they were fertile and would bear healthy offspring. Invariably, that meant picking females who displayed the unmistakable signs of youth, such as clear, smooth, unwrinkled skin; a firm body; and shiny hair. Gray locks on a woman were a physical cue that her youth—more specifically, her fertility—had passed.

Our female ancestors had different standards. Gray hair on a male wasn't a liability. In fact, it was a plus. Those steely locks meant that he had resources, power, and status—the things that women have always needed to rear their babies. To a female, a gray-haired male would be able to provide for and protect her and her offspring.

Of course, we no longer choose mates purely on the basis of their physical attributes. Our "selection process" is much more sophisticated. We look for a mate for love, not just procreation. And yet, in that small Stone Age part of men's brains, a woman's gray locks still signal age, while in the woman's mind, a man's signal status.

*Expert consulted*
*Helen Fisher, Ph.D.*
*Research associate in the department*
*of anthropology*
*Rutgers University, New Brunswick, New Jersey*
*Author of* Anatomy of Love

**Restore hair from the inside.** A good deep conditioner fills hair shafts with protein so that hair repels moisture better. Look for a product that contains wheat germ or soybean protein. Apply it twice a month to start, then cut back to once a month as your hair improves. (If you color your hair, avoid using hot-oil treatments and other heated deep conditioners for at least 10 days afterward. Otherwise, the color will fade or turn brassy.)

**Add gel.** Molding gel seals out excessive moisture and protects against environmental elements. Work the gel into sections of wet hair, starting at the nape of your neck and moving up toward the center of your head. Repeat, each time sliding your fingers closer to your ears. Finish with the forehead and hairline area.

**Put away the blow-dryer.** After shampooing and conditioning, squeeze excess water from your hair using a towel. Then allow your hair to air-dry.

## Gray Hair

If you wonder when your hair will start turning gray (if it hasn't already), take a look at Mom and Dad. Graying is hereditary, and there's no avoiding it. Everyone eventually goes gray, as individual hair follicles stop producing pigment.

Surprisingly, only about one-third of all women opt for the cover-up. The rest let nature make the choice. But even Mother Nature has some secrets to help give gray hair a youthful sheen.

your scalp. Leave the detangler on for two to three minutes so that your hair has a chance to absorb the moisture. Then rinse, leaving a little of the detangler in.

**Rinse with sage or rosemary.** To gently darken brown or black hair that's showing signs of gray, use a rinse made from sage or rosemary. Add between two teaspoons and one tablespoon of either dried herb to a cup of boiling water. Let the liquid cool to a comfortable temperature, strain out the herb, and pour the liquid over your hair after shampooing. Don't rinse it out. Repeat each time you wash your hair until you've covered the gray.

**Add nettle and walnut to the mix.** For auburn, brown, or medium to dark gray hair, use a coloring made with nettle and black walnut hulls (available at health food stores or by mail-order catalogs). To prepare the coloring, boil eight cups of water and add one-quarter cup each of dried sage, rosemary, and nettle; one-half cup of black walnut hulls; and two black tea bags. Allow the mixture to steep for three hours, then strain out the herbs and walnut hulls and add two teaspoons of sweet almond or olive oil. Keep the mixture refrigerated until you're ready to use it. After you wash and rinse your hair, slip on a pair of rubber gloves and work one-half cup of the mixture through your hair, being careful not to get it on your forehead, neck, and temples. Wait a minute or so before towel-drying your hair. Use a dark towel so that the stains won't show.

## Oily Hair

The term *oily hair* is something of a misnomer. The oil comes not from your hair but from your scalp. Like the rest of your skin, your scalp has sebaceous glands. They secrete sebum, a mixture of fatty acids that keeps your scalp from drying out. In some people, the sebaceous glands churn out so much sebum that each hair shaft becomes slickly coated and weighted down. Hair appears greasy, flat, and lifeless.

Sebum production is regulated by hormones.

Women who have oily hair often find that the problem literally dries up after they go through menopause, when their hormone levels decline. In the meantime, you can control greasiness by following this advice.

**Wash in the A.M.** You work up a sweat while you sleep. So by morning, even hair shampooed just before bedtime looks oily and matted.

**Stir up your own shampoo.** Add four drops of rosemary essential oil and four drops of lavender essential oil to two ounces of any unscented shampoo. Shake to mix well, then use a quarter-size dollop to wash your hair. Rosemary and lavender tone your scalp and add shine. The essential oils are available in health food stores and bath-and-beauty shops.

**Trade off.** Alternate your regular shampoo with a clarifying shampoo, which removes oil from the hair shaft as well as from your scalp. Check labels for a product that is high in cleaning agents such as sodium lauryl sulfate and low in conditioning agents such as lanolin.

**Rinse with vinegar.** Vinegar reduces soap and hard-water residues to make your hair soft and shiny. Mix one cup of vinegar with one cup of water, then pour the solution over your hair as a final rinse. Vinegar's aroma quickly fades.

**Curtail conditioning.** Most conditioners and styling products contain ingredients that weigh hair down, the last thing you need if your hair is oily.

**Cut back on brushing.** The more you brush, the more you spread oil from your scalp to your hair.

## Split Ends

What with blow-dryers, curling irons, and other heated styling appliances, there is no end to the times we end up with split ends. The intense temperature causes hair strands to crack at the tip and split up the shaft.

Keeping up with your hair cuts is the easiest way to make split ends disappear. Just make sure that the stylist is using sharp scissors. Dull scissors can actually cause split ends. If you tend to have long spells between cuts, here's what to do.

**Get in the thick of things.** Look for a shampoo and a conditioner that contain waxes or other thickening agents.

**Allow hair to air-dry.** The intense heat from blow-drying causes split ends.

**Turn down the temp.** If you must use a blow-dryer or another heated appliance, first spray your damp hair with a thermal styling conditioner. And set the appliance on the lowest setting to minimize heat damage.

## Thinning

Everyone sheds between 50 and 100 hairs per day. The average hair has a life span of three to six years, entering a resting stage of about three months before falling out. Then a new hair sprouts in its place from the same roots.

Sometimes, though, the hair growth cycle gets messed up, causing hundreds of hairs to fall out per day. In women, hormonal changes brought on by pregnancy, menopause, and the use of oral contraceptives can alter hair-growing conditions. So can rapid weight loss, iron deficiency, serious illness, and extreme physical stress (such as childbirth).

Some women even have a genetic predisposition to hair loss, just as some men do. It can come from either parent.

If you seem to be losing more hair than normal, see your doctor. She can examine you for an underlying medical problem and prescribe proper treatment. Then use these measures to care for your remaining hair and discourage more loss.

**Baby your mane.** Wash your hair with a baby shampoo, lathering up only once and rubbing your scalp gently. After rinsing, spray your hair with a detangling conditioner.

**Pull the plug.** Allow your hair to dry naturally whenever possible. If you must use a blow-dryer, set it on low.

**Wait while wet.** Wait until your hair is completely dry before combing or brushing. Otherwise, it can stretch and break. And never tease your hair, which also causes breakage.

**Get more B$_6$.** Vitamin B$_6$ seems to slow the rate of hair loss in some people. Take 100 milligrams a day in supplement form.

**Mine for iron.** Iron deficiency can contribute to hair loss, so eat one to two servings of iron-rich foods every day. Good sources of the mineral include lean red meat, Cream of Wheat cereal, tofu, and broccoli.

**Put protein on your plate.** Without adequate protein, your body can't make new hair to replace what has fallen out. So eat two three- to four-ounce servings of chicken, fish, or other lean protein every day.

# Sweet Relief for Feet

If you happen to visit a podiatrist's office any time soon, take a look around the waiting room while you're there. Chances are that women will outnumber men four to one.

That's because women have four times as many foot problems as men. And women account for 90 percent of all foot surgeries. Not that our feet are any different from men's, structurally speaking. We just seem to have a propensity for squeezing them into shoes that are too high, too pointy, and too tight.

"Women's footwear has long been designed for style rather than function," observes Pamela Colman, D.P.M., director of health affairs at the American Podiatric Medical Association. "Almost every common foot problem that you can think of—blisters, corns, calluses—results from poorly shaped, poorly constructed, ill-fitting shoes."

Women over age 65 are especially prone to foot problems because they've worn pointed-toe high heels for most of their lives. They have 3½ times more calluses and corns and 13 times more bunions than men of the same age.

## Shoe Sense

The easiest way to keep your feet out of the doctor's office is to wear sensible shoes. Thankfully, many of us are getting the message. "Maybe it's because athletic shoes are 'in' right now, but I've noticed that more women are choosing footwear more for comfort than for style," Dr. Colman says.

How can you be sure that you're getting the best shoes for your feet? Dr. Colman offers this brief buyer's guide.

❧ Shop for shoes in the latter part of the day, when your feet have swollen to their maximum.

❧ Have both feet measured for length and width. "It's not at all unusual to have one foot be a little longer than the other," Dr. Colman says. If you do, fit shoes to the longer foot.

❧ Always try shoes on. "Manufacturers use different lasts, or forms, to make shoes," Dr. Colman explains. "So even though your foot measures a size 6, you may not be a size 6 in every brand of shoe."

## THE PRICE OF PRETTY FEET

The perfect pedicure—soft, smooth skin and painted toes—may look great in sandals. But once you fling them off, you'll be hop, hop, hopping across the sand to escape the heat of the burning sun.

While many women are willing to pay a pretty price for creams and lotions for pretty feet, the calluses they are buffing away are making their feet (especially when going shoeless) more vulnerable to aches and pain.

"Calluses are nothing more than thickened skin caused by excessive pressure on part of the foot," explains Ellen J. Sobel, D.P.M., Ph.D., associate professor in the division of orthopedic sciences at the New York College of Podiatric Medicine in New York City. "They're not especially attractive but may offer protection."

For example, if you frequently wear high-heeled shoes, calluses help cushion those parts of your feet that bear your body weight. The same is true if you have high arches, flat feet, or some other structural problem. For women who are on their feet all day, calluses are the cushions that keep their feet from aching.

What's more, while callus-removing products seem harmless enough, they can make matters worse if they're not used properly. "The patients I see usually leave them on too long," Dr. Sobel says. "They're only supposed to be left on overnight. They can burn the skin; it actually turns white."

Still, Dr. Sobel believes that callus-removing products have their place. "Provided they're applied according to the label directions, they can be especially effective for very thick calluses on the heels or under the metatarsals (the bones that connect the toes to the midfoot)," she says. "But really, if your callus doesn't cause any pain or discomfort, I'd recommend leaving it alone."

And if you have diabetes, never try to remove a callus on your own. The decreased sensitivity in your feet can make a minor problem much worse. See a podiatrist.

* Buy the pair that feels most comfortable when you try them on. Don't expect to break them in.

Buying the right shoes is crucial, but it's only part of the equation. Dr. Colman suggests adding these strategies to your foot-care routine.

* Get rid of worn-out shoes. How can you tell? Set them on a table or on another flat surface. If they're not perfectly level—if either shoe tilts in or out—they're no longer supporting your feet as they should be.

* Wear flip-flops rather than walking barefoot. Otherwise, you are exposing your feet not just to viruses and fungi but also to foreign objects.

* After bathing, be sure to dry between your toes. This area is a haven for moisture-loving, disease-causing microorganisms.

* After bathing, massage your feet with a moisturizing lotion.

* When giving yourself a pedicure, cut your toenails straight across and then gently file the edges with an emery board. You'll minimize your chances of getting an ingrown toenail.

All the above strategies can help keep your feet healthy and problem-free. But if you are bothered by a specific foot problem, read on for expert-recommended tips.

* Look for shoes made from breathable material, like leather or canvas.

* Avoid styles with pointy toes or heels higher than two inches.

## Blisters

Combine shoes that don't fit properly with almost any activity that has you on your feet, and you'll probably end up with a blister.

Although painful, a blister serves an important purpose. The fluid sealed inside keeps the skin moist and helps it heal. Ideally, the blister should be left intact to protect the skin against infection. But if it does open, that's okay, as long as you take extra care to keep the wound clean.

To baby your unbroken blister and speed the healing process, follow this advice.

**Alleviate pain with aloe.** A popular remedy for burns, aloe also heals blisters, thanks to its anti-inflammatory and antibiotic properties. Just smear some gel on the blister and cover it with gauze or a sterile bandage.

**Be blister-free with comfrey.** The herb comfrey contains the compound allantoin, which can help heal wounds. You can buy comfrey cream in health food stores. Or you can make a poultice from the herb by following this recipe: Cut up a handful of dried comfrey leaves (available at health food stores), cover them with boiling water, and let steep for 10 minutes. Allow to cool, then strain the leaves from the water. Gently squeeze the leaves to remove any excess water. Put the moistened herb on a piece of gauze and place the gauze on top of the blister with the leaves on top of the gauze. Cover with another piece of gauze and secure in place with an elastic bandage for at least 20 minutes. Do this twice daily.

**Feel relief with calendula.** A combination of the herb calendula

REAL-LIFE SCENARIO

### Dressed to Kill: Her Feet or Her Career?

**Donna's feet are a mess. At 39, she has corns that are so painful that she hates to put on her shoes in the morning. When the corns get really hard, she uses a pumice stone to gently rub them off. But they keep coming back. When she gets home at night after a long day on her feet, her feet ache and swell so much that she has to hobble around in slippers. She tried switching to dressy flats instead of heels for work, but that made her arches hurt. She loves her job in retail sales but is thinking of switching to phone sales so that she doesn't have to spend so much time on her feet. Is there anything more she can do to save her feet—and her career?**

Donna has a classic case of professional woman's shoe syndrome. And it's not uncommon in women who have to spend all day on their feet.

For starters, she should see a podiatrist. She may have a bone or structural problem.

In the meantime, there's plenty that she can do to pamper her feet. Each night, she should rub her feet with vitamin E cream or oil, which will soothe the skin and lessen the pain. A foot soak in cool water after work will also help bring the swelling down as will simply elevating her feet.

Most important, Donna needs to change her taste in shoes. She needs to go for a wider, squarer toebox to give her toes room to wiggle throughout the day.

Donna can also invest in a pair of arch supports to keep her standing tall after a long day on the sales floor. An over-the-counter set may just do the trick; if not, a podiatrist can fit Donna with a pair prescription-made for her.

Finally, doing these two little foot-strengthening exercises as often as possible will help her go the extra mile: She can drop a washcloth on the floor and pick it up with her toes. And then roll the arch of each foot over a can of soup or vegetables that has cooled in the refrigerator.

**Expert consulted**
*Kathleen Stone, D.P.M.*
*Podiatrist at Thunderbird Footcare*
*Glendale, Arizona*

and vitamin E can speed the healing of blisters by reducing inflammation. Mix equal parts calendula oil and vitamin E oil and spread it on the blister. Calendula and vitamin E oil are available in drugstores and health food stores.

If you don't have actual vitamin E oil on hand, poke open a vitamin E capsule with a pin and squeeze out the capsule's contents.

**Give it air.** You want to protect the blistered area with a bandage while you're wearing shoes. But when you can, take off your shoes and bandage and allow the blister to breathe. Air helps it heal faster.

**Pop with precision.** If a blister becomes too uncomfortable, go ahead and pop it—the right way. Sterilize a needle by holding it to a small flame. Make several small holes at the sides of the blister. (Don't prick the blister only once; it may quickly reseal.) Allow the liquid to flow out of the holes. Leave the top flap of skin in place to protect the wound. Apply an antibiotic liquid over the area and cover it with gauze to eliminate bacteria that could cause infection. Change the gauze twice a day. If you have diabetes, you should not attempt this without consulting with your doctor.

## Bunions

Does your foot resemble a triangle, with the tip of your big toe or little toe angling inward and your joint jutting outward? If so, you have a bunion. And it probably hurts.

While shoes can aggravate bunions, they don't actually cause them. You inherit the shape of your feet from your ancestors.

## CRUEL SHOES

In China, where petite feet were once considered beautiful, young girls' feet were bound so that they'd remain only a few inches long. Though such a custom is now considered barbaric, some podiatrists would argue that modern women practice their own version of foot binding, thanks to their penchant for too-tight, too-pointed, high-heeled shoes.

"Many women prefer high heels because they think heels look more appropriate with professional clothes," says Pamela Colman, D.P.M., director of health affairs at the American Podiatric Medical Association. "But the majority of shoes fit so poorly that, over the course of a lifetime, they slowly deform the feet."

Among common problems are blisters, calluses, corns, hammertoes, neuromas, and bunions.

**When you wear shoes with heels higher than two inches, all of your body weight shifts forward onto the balls of your feet and your toes. The constant pressure, especially on your toes, can lead to an array of foot problems.**

Many women can live with the discomfort of bunions. But sometimes the pain becomes so severe that simple physical activity such as walking becomes difficult. In such cases, surgery may provide the only real relief.

That said, you can do a lot on your own to keep your foot comfortable and prevent a bunion from getting worse. Start with these strategies.

**Put your bunion on ice.** Your bunion may be inflamed if it feels hot and swollen. You can cool it down with an ice pack wrapped in a damp cloth. Apply it to your bunion for 10 to 15 minutes.

**Flat and low-heeled shoes with a generous toebox area evenly distribute your body weight between the balls of your feet and your heels. Your toes are free to help you keep your balance, uninhibited by pain, irritation, or swelling.**

**High heels often have pointed toeboxes. Over time, your toes assume the triangular shape of the toebox, setting the stage for hammertoes, neuromas, and bunions.**

**Pick pineapple.** Pineapple contains the compound bromelain, which acts as an anti-inflammatory to reduce the swelling and pain associated with bunions. Simply wipe the inside of a small piece of the peel from a fresh pineapple directly over your bunion. Or take 250 to 500 milligrams of pure bromelain in capsule form three times a day. You can find the capsules in health food stores and in some drugstores.

**Buy new shoes.** Although a change of footwear won't get rid of bunions, it may make them less painful. Wear athletic shoes as often as you can. They provide excellent comfort and

support for feet with bunions. If you must wear dress shoes, choose a pair that has no more than $1\frac{1}{2}$-inch heels.

## Calluses

Like a blister, a callus results from the friction created when shoe rubs against skin.

Generally, a callus will become a problem only when it grows big enough to become a source of pressure and discomfort. Still, if you have one, you'd probably like to see it disappear. These self-care measures can help.

**Put pumice to work.** Use a pumice stone, which is actually volcanic glass, to rub off the dead skin of the callus and reveal the smoother skin underneath. You can buy pumice stones in drugstores, beauty supply stores, and some health food stores.

To begin, soak your feet in plain lukewarm water for 5 to 10 minutes to soften the callus. Then gently rub the stone back and forth across the callus. (If you have diabetes, decreased circulation, or decreased sensitivity, talk to your podiatrist before you attempt this.)

**Let E do the healing.** After rubbing the callus with a pumice stone, apply a vitamin E cream or oil. Vitamin E penetrates well and keeps the skin soft.

**Use the correct lotion.** Lotions made with urea can help prevent a hard callus by getting rid of dead skin and stopping its buildup. Look for them in drugstores and large supermarkets.

## Corns

Corns form the same way calluses do, as layers of skin build up to protect points on the feet against constant rubbing by ill-fitting shoes. The main difference between the two is that corns sprout on top of or in between toes, while calluses develop primarily on the heels and soles.

If a corn becomes thick enough to put pressure on nerves, it can hurt. But you don't have to live with the discomfort. Try these self-care strategies instead.

**Change your lacing.** If you have a corn on top of your toe, run the lace of your shoe from one bottom eyelet to the top eyelet on the opposite side. Weave the lace through the remaining eyelets, alternating from side to side. Tying your shoe in this way lifts the toebox, so your toes have more room.

**Cushion the corn.** To lessen the pain of a corn located between your toes, cover it with a tuft of lamb's wool, available in drugstores.

**Rub in castor oil.** Castor oil softens corns and makes them less painful and easier to file down with a pumice stone. Massage your feet with the oil every night.

**File away the offender.** Soak your feet in warm water, then use a pumice stone to remove the hardened skin. Don't try to file away the entire corn in one sitting; you'll only irritate the skin. Instead, work at the corn a little bit each night until it's gone.

## Foot Odor

Like other body parts, your feet perspire. But the perspiration itself doesn't make your feet smell. Rather, moisture that gets trapped in your shoes enables bacteria to grow, which create the offending odor. Here's what to do.

**Roll away the odor.** For a quick fix, apply your underarm deodorant to the bottom of your feet. It will fight bacterial odor, although it won't control wetness.

**Massage with essential oils.** Lavender and tea tree oils are potent antimicrobials, so they'll kill the bacteria that are causing foot odor. The oils smell good, too. You can buy them in health food stores and bath-and-beauty shops. Apply one of these oils (dilute 15 drops in a carrier oil) at bedtime, rubbing enough into your feet to coat the skin. Slip on socks to protect your sheets. Repeat the treatment for at least four consecutive nights.

**Drown the stench.** Soak your feet in one of the following solutions for 15 to 20 minutes once or twice a day.

- Epsom salts. Add one-half cup Epsom salts to a quart of warm water.
- Tea. Steep a few regular black tea bags in hot water, then add some cool water so that the tea is a lukewarm temperature. Black tea has tannins, which help absorb moisture.
- Vinegar. Add one-half cup white vinegar to a quart of warm water.

**Pamper your footwear.** The insides of shoes are dark and damp, an environment in which bacteria thrive. To discourage microbes from making themselves at home in your footwear, follow this advice.

- Alternate your shoes on a daily basis.
- Don't keep your shoes in a closed, dark place like a locker.
- If you exercise daily, alternate two pairs of athletic shoes.

## Hammertoes

The name is apropos because hammertoes are caused by beating up our feet by—what else?—wearing tight, pointed-toe shoes.

The shape of the shoe's toebox forces both sides of the foot (the big toe and/or the pinky toe) to turn inward, crowding the other toes. Sometimes a toe can get squeezed so much that it curls into an arched position. That's a hammertoe.

If you have a hammertoe, surgery can straighten it. But that should be a last resort. Before you do anything so drastic, try these strategies.

**Use your marbles.** Pick up 20 marbles with your toes three times a day. This exercise strengthens the tendons in your feet, so the hammertoe stays flexible.

**Lend some support.** A device called a crest pad can keep a hammertoe from curling under. The pad—actually a tapered foam cushion—is placed under the toes and attached to the top of the foot. You can buy crest pads in medical supply stores.

**Find accommodating footwear.** Make sure that your shoe has a toebox that is high enough and wide enough to allow enough room for your hammertoe.

## Neuromas

If walking a certain way causes a quick, sharp shot of pain that could send you through the roof, chances are that you have a neuroma. A neu-

---

### REPAIRING AN INGROWN NAIL

Toenails are made to be as tough as . . . well, nails. So when a toenail happens to dig into the delicate flesh of a tender tootsie, the pain can be pretty intense.

An ingrown toenail usually occurs for one of two reasons. You may have trimmed your nail in such a way that it started growing into the surrounding skin. Or you may have worn a pair of too-tight shoes that squeezed your toes together, pushing nail into skin.

If you have an ingrown toenail, you should start treating it as soon as possible to prevent it from becoming infected. Here's what doctors suggest you do.

1. Add one to two tablespoons of salt to a quart of lukewarm water. Soak your feet for 15 to 20 minutes. This softens the nail and the skin around it. It also helps fight infection.

2. With a rounded toothpick, carefully lift the edge of the ingrown toenail as much as you can tolerate. Then slide a small piece of gauze or cotton under the nail where it's digging into your skin. This will encourage the nail to grow out and over the gauze or cotton. If you are unable to do this step, see your doctor.

**The tools for curing an ingrown nail include tweezers, a rounded toothpick, and a small piece of cotton. Insert the cotton under the nail as shown.**

3. Change the gauze or cotton every day until your toe heals.

While your toe is on the mend, keep it uncovered as much as possible. Take off your shoes and socks or stockings when you're at home, and wear sandals when you can. Also, don't bandage your toe. If you notice any redness, pus, or swelling or if the toe feels more tender after a couple of days, see your doctor.

roma is an enlarged nerve that has a tendency to get in the way of the tiny bones on the ball of your foot (usually around your fourth toe). Pain lets you know when it happens.

If the pain is unbearable, your doctor may recommend cortisone injections, padding, or even surgery. Fortunately, most neuromas can be managed with sensible self-care. Here's what to do.

**Treat your feet.** When the pain of a neuroma has your feet in a bind, give them a rest and try elevating them. Also, walk barefoot around the house as much as possible.

**Provide padding.** A ball-of-the-foot support pad placed in your shoe will reduce pressure on the affected nerve. You can buy the pads in drugstores.

**Size up your shoes.** Wearing a shoe with a low heel (no more than two inches) and a wide enough and high enough toebox will alleviate the pressure on your toes. And that will keep your neuroma from hurting.

## Sore Feet

The average woman puts approximately 500 pounds of pressure on her feet just by walking. Multiply that by about 10,000 steps a day, and the stage is set for sore feet.

**Put icing on the ache.** To reduce inflammation, apply ice to your feet for 15 to 20 minutes once or twice a day. Wrap the ice in a towel so that it doesn't touch your skin. Continue the treatment for two or three consecutive days.

**Play toe tennis.** Stand with your foot on a tennis ball. Working from the center of your heel, move the ball down either side of your heel toward the ball of your foot. Massaging your foot in this way relaxes the muscles and tissues in the arch of your foot and spreads the metatarsals, the bones in the ball of your foot.

**Roll a can for relief.** To soothe an aching arch, roll your bare foot over a can of frozen juice concentrate for 5 to 10 minutes. Wrap the can in a towel so that it doesn't touch your skin. The massage helps loosen tense tissues, while the cold helps reduce inflammation.

**Stretch out tension.** If you have pain between your toes or in the ball of your foot, try this exercise. Lace your fingers between your toes and stretch your toes apart very gently. This exercise helps keep your toes flexible and gives the connective tissue in your feet a good stretch.

**Find your marbles.** Using your toes, pick up marbles off of the floor and drop them into a container. Or place small objects like pencils or corks between your toes and then squeeze for five seconds.

# Plenty of Reasons to Smile

A passionate kiss between lovers. A hearty laugh between friends. A tender smile between mother and child. For some of life's simplest pleasures, we have our mouths to thank. So let's give them the respect they deserve.

"The best thing a woman can do to keep the inside of her mouth healthy is brush and floss regularly," says Esther Rubin, D.D.S., a dentist in New York City. "Proper self-care can prevent most, if not all, teeth and gum problems."

Poor dental hygiene can lead to trouble down the line, starting with gingivitis and ending with periodontitis, serious gum deterioration that can lead to tooth loss if it is not treated in time. To nip tooth problems in the bud, here's what to do.

## Gingivitis

Gingivitis is a form of gum disease caused when dental plaque (a gluelike film of bacteria, food, and saliva) invades the warm and inviting crevasses at and below the gum line. There it hardens into tartar (sometimes called calculus), triggering inflammation and infection.

Left untreated, gingivitis can lead to periodontitis, a condition characterized by severely receding gums and, ultimately, destruction of the jawbone, which anchors your teeth in place. But gingivitis doesn't have to get nearly that far. Combine the following strategies with regular brushing and flossing to combat gingivitis and keep your gums in the pink. If your gums continue to bleed each time you brush, make an appointment to see your dentist.

**Make your own herbal toothpaste.** Mix one tablespoon of the herb goldenseal in dried form with enough water to form a paste. Then brush your teeth as you normally would. Goldenseal, which is available in health food stores, can help heal inflamed, diseased gums. (If you are allergic to plants in the daisy family, goldenseal may cause an allergic reaction.)

**Brush with baking soda.** Mix baking soda with enough hydrogen peroxide to form a paste. With your toothbrush, gently rub the mixture onto your gums. Leave it on for a few minutes, then rinse.

**Sip a soothing tea.** Add two tablespoons of the dried herb anise and two tablespoons of

## "I Cured My Gingivitis and Kept My Smile"

*Henrietta Johnson, 43, the owner of a pet service in New York City, was in danger of losing her teeth before she used natural remedies to turn the situation around. Here's her story.*

When I was a kid, I had great teeth—not a cavity in my mouth. Then, when I was around 19 or 20, I started getting a barrage of cavities. My gums were in trouble, too. I'd eat an apple and they'd bleed—a classic sign of gingivitis. At that time, I was brushing my teeth once a day and I wasn't flossing at all.

Then a few years ago during a routine dental visit, my dentist found a 10-millimeter pocket between my back lower molar and the surrounding gum. Smaller pockets were forming around other teeth as well. Basically, I was in danger of my gums eventually loosening their hold on my teeth.

My dentist suggested gum surgery to repair the largest pocket. I said, "There has to be something else I can do." I was determined to heal my gums on my own.

I started brushing my teeth twice a day with Weleda Salt Toothpaste. I still do. It doesn't contain saccharin, and the salt helps tighten the gums. At night, I add two drops of tea tree oil to my toothpaste. (Essential oils can be toxic if swallowed, so don't use this on children.) It's a natural—and powerful—antiseptic, and it kills the bacteria that damage the gums. I floss twice a day as well. I take coenzyme $Q_{10}$ every day. It boosts the body's immunity and is an excellent treatment for gum disease. Finally, I get my teeth cleaned four times a year instead of the recommended two times.

After following this regimen for a year, my gums improved dramatically. They don't hurt, they don't bleed, they don't itch, and they're not swollen. And that 10-millimeter pocket? According to my dentist, it actually shrank to 8 millimeters. Those other pockets got smaller, too. If I keep up the routine—keep those pockets clean—I believe that my gums will be okay. And best of all, I avoided surgery.

dried sage (both sold in health food stores) to one cup of freshly boiled water. Allow the herbs to steep for 10 minutes, then strain the tea and drink up. Repeat as needed to relieve sore gums.

**Be generous with garlic.** Garlic is nature's antibiotic. It helps to fight plaque-forming bacteria, which means that they are less likely to set up shop in your mouth. You can increase your intake of fresh garlic simply by adding it to most of your meals. Worried about garlic breath? Then take supplements instead—250 milligrams a day.

**Take your Q.** Coenzyme $Q_{10}$ is a natural compound that may help treat gingivitis and can promote healthy gum tissue by increasing the flow of oxygen to cells. You will find coenzyme $Q_{10}$ supplements in health food stores.

**Sing for high C.** Vitamin C can help gum tissue resist the bacterial onslaught that leads to gingivitis. Take 500 milligrams three times a day.

*Note:* Some people develop diarrhea when taking high doses of vitamin C. If this happens, cut back your dosage to a tolerable level.

## Tooth Discoloration

Beginning in their late thirties, many women notice that their once pearly whites are taking on a different hue. Teeth naturally lose some of their outermost layer—the enamel—over the years. And because the material beneath the enamel is darker, your bright smile will begin to fade.

Unless you have a calcium deficiency, which will require a doctor's intervention, tooth discoloration is essentially a cosmetic problem. The following tips will discourage stains and spiff up your smile.

**Whiten wisely.** As a natural alternative to home bleaching kits, which can irritate gums, look in your health food store for a product called Peelu. It's a whitener made from tree root extract and sold as a toothpaste and a powder.

**Chew gum as a chaser.** After drinking coffee or tea, chew a stick of sugarless gum. This stimulates the production of saliva to help wash away the beverage's residues before they stain.

**Sip water to stop stains.** Out of gum? Then take a swig of water and swish it around your mouth. Water is enough to clean your teeth and prevent stains from building up.

## Tooth Grinding

Most women who grind their teeth don't even know until some else tells them about it. That's because tooth grinding (also called bruxism) often occurs during sleep.

Tooth grinding can lead to a variety of problems, including headaches, jaw pain, tooth sensitivity, and temporomandibular disorder, in which the hinges of the jaw malfunction. If you routinely have tooth or face pain when you wake up, see a dentist.

### RAGING HORMONES, BLEEDING GUMS?

You brush. You floss. And still, your gums bleed. What's the deal?

You're a woman.

Menstruation, pregnancy, menopause, and birth control pills all cause hormonal changes that reduce the ability of a woman's gum tissues to fight the bacteria that cause gingivitis, says Barbara A. Rich, D.D.S., a dentist in Cherry Hill, New Jersey.

This hormonal roller-coaster can decrease your gums' ability to become tough or less penetrable (what dentists call keratinization), one of the barriers that prevent bacteria from invading and damaging gum tissue, says Dr. Rich.

Bleeding gums can also signal that a woman's physical and emotional health is out of balance, says Andrea Brockman, D.D.S., board member of the Holistic Dental Association in practice at the Valley Green Center for Holistic Dentistry in Philadelphia. Chronic stress, poor diet, and inadequate sleep can weaken the immune system, allowing gum-damaging bacteria to thrive.

To avoid bleeding gums, you should cut back on red meat, sugar, processed foods, caffeine, and alcohol, says Dr. Brockman. "They can make saliva extremely acidic, and bacteria thrive in an acidic environment." Avoid smoking and eat more fish, whole grains, and raw fruits and vegetables. Also, get sufficient refreshing sleep, aerobic exercise, and fresh air and practice some form of stress-reduction technique.

For already sore gums, turn to tea tree, lavender, eucalyptus, or peppermint essential oils to inhibit the growth of bacteria and speed away infection, says Dr. Brockman. If you use a pulsating irrigation device such as a Water Pik or Hydro Floss, add up to five drops of one of these oils in five ounces of distilled water to the reservoir. "The oils will penetrate and stay in the gingival tissues," says Dr. Brockman.

Or, mix up to five drops of one of the oils with a few ounces of distilled water and swish it around in your mouth two or three times a day. (Essential oils can be toxic if swallowed, so don't use this on children.)

Fortunately, you can do things while you're awake to soothe a painful jaw and break the tooth-grinding habit. Here's what dentists recommend.

**Get immediate relief with heat.** Soak a towel in warm water, wring it out, and wrap it around a hot water bottle. Apply this compress to your face for 15 to 20 minutes, frequently checking your skin to make sure that it's not getting burned.

**Sip herbal tea before snoozing.** Considering a nightcap to help you relax? Some research suggests that drinking alcohol before going to bed can exacerbate tooth grinding. Have a cup of herbal tea instead.

**Follow the dots.** Go to your nearest office supply store and buy a sheet or two of orange dot stickers. Paste them everywhere: on your mirror, your dashboard, and your refrigerator door. Every time you see one, take it as your cue to separate your teeth. This simple trick discourages tooth grinding.

## Tooth Sensitivity

Its lightning bolt of pain can turn a sweet experience, like sipping an ice-cold glass of lemonade, sour real fast.

If you have a sensitive tooth, you may decide to deal with it by avoiding whatever triggers your pain. That's fine for a temporary fix. You really need to have the tooth checked out by your dentist to determine what's wrong. In the meantime, these self-care measures can minimize your discomfort.

**Pass the jelly.** Petroleum jelly doesn't feel or taste very good inside

## BRUSHING AND FLOSSING: DO IT RIGHT

You've been brushing your teeth all your life, so why would you need instructions on something so elementary? Because you probably aren't doing it right.

"A lot of women think that they're doing a great job of cleaning their teeth, but they've never had instruction and they're not using proper technique," observes Esther Rubin, D.D.S., a dentist in New York City.

Thoroughly brushing your teeth takes at least three minutes—not the 51 seconds that most women allow. Brushing *and* flossing are important because they prevent the formation of plaque, a sticky film of bacteria, mucus, and food particles that coats teeth and eventually causes cavities and gingivitis (swollen, bleeding gums).

Dentists agree that the easiest, most effective way to keep your teeth and gums healthy is to practice good oral hygiene. To do it right, follow these three steps, then finish by brushing the surface of your tongue, which can harbor bacteria and contribute to bad breath.

**1. Position the brush at a 45-degree angle to your gum line. Use short back-and-forth strokes to clean the outside of your teeth and then the inside.**

**2. Brush the chewing surfaces of your teeth.**

**3. Clean the inside of your front teeth by holding the brush perpendicular to your gums. Move the brush from the gum toward the biting edge—up on your lower teeth, down on your upper teeth.**

Ideally, your teeth should be brushed five times a day: in the morning, at bedtime, and after each meal. At least one of those sessions should be followed by flossing. "Personally, I think that flossing is the best investment a person can make in terms of dental health," Dr. Rubin says. "Proper flossing can save your teeth."

Be sure to pick the right floss for you. If you have rough fillings or if your teeth are close together, waxed floss works best. Unwaxed floss is thinner than waxed, but it also frays more readily. If your teeth are widely spaced or if you have a hard time flossing, dental tape is a good choice.

To practice proper flossing, follow these five steps.

1. Tear off a strand of floss about 18 inches long. Wrap the ends around the middle fingers of both hands until just 6 to 8 inches of floss is exposed.

2. Pinch the floss between the thumb and index finger of one hand. With the index finger of your other hand, guide about one inch of floss between your teeth.

3. Use a back-and-forth motion as you gently slide the floss up and down between your teeth.

4. Curve the floss around the base of each tooth. Gently move the floss back and forth beneath the gum line.

5. To remove the floss, use the same back-and-forth motion to bring it up and away from your teeth. Never snap or force the floss, or you might bruise delicate gum tissue.

your mouth, but it will quiet a sensitive tooth on a short-term basis. Simply apply petroleum jelly to the tooth.

**Extend an olive branch.** If tooth sensitivity results from an abrasion or erosion along the gum line, olive oil can help. Warm the oil by pouring a small amount into a saucepan and heating it until it starts to smoke. Dampen a cotton swab in the oil, then wave the swab in the air briefly to cool it off. Dry the affected tooth with a tissue or cotton ball and then dab the warm oil on your gum line a couple of times. Repeat as needed. (One treatment may last for months.)

**Take a hard look at soft drinks.** If you're drinking enough colas and root beers to float an armada, cut back. The darker sodas have high levels of phosphoric acid, which pulls calcium out of your body—and your teeth— like crazy.

**Switch to a softer brush.** A tooth can become sensitive because of overly aggressive brushing, especially with a brush that has hard bristles. This combination can push back the gum and expose the root surface. Use a toothbrush with softer bristles and adapt a gentler brushing technique.

## Chapped Lips

Your lips do a remarkable job of keeping your teeth protected, and in doing so, they take their own form of abuse. For all the wear and tear that they endure, lips are remarkably unprotected. They lack the natural oils that keep the rest of your skin supple. They also lack melanin, the pigment that

## WOMEN ASK WHY

### If they're supposed to be wisdom teeth, why is the dentist so eager to pull them?

Wisdom teeth, or third molars, are the last teeth to develop and appear in the mouth. They are so named because they usually appear during our late teens or early twenties—what has been dubbed the age of wisdom.

Dentists usually yank them because most of us don't have room for them in our mouths. And many dentists believe that if we get those big guys pulled before they're fully formed, we're much wiser for it. Saving a set of wisdom teeth "just in case" there's room could set you up for problems later in life. Here's why.

A wisdom tooth left to its own devices may become partially trapped, or impacted, under your 12-year molars (so called because that's the age at which they usually appear), where it can grow any which way. Food can easily get packed around partially impacted (partially grown in) wisdom teeth and the molar next to it, possibly causing an abscess or gum disease.

So why did nature give us a set of teeth too big to accommodate? Apparently, they served a purpose long ago. Evolution tells us that in the past, humans had bigger jaws, which were needed to gnaw at food before proper utensils were invented.

*Expert consulted*
*Heidi Hausauer, D.D.S.*
*Spokesperson for the Academy of General*
*    Dentistry*
*University of the Pacific*
*Castro Valley, California*

A few days of TLC—tender lip care—is all you should need to restore the wetness to your whistle. Here's what to do. (If you have severely cracked lips, see your doctor. You may need a prescription preparation.)

**Smear on the old standby.** For chapped lips, nothing works better than petroleum jelly.

**Thumb your nose at dryness.** If you have oily skin and you're outdoors with no lip balm handy, run your finger along the side of your nose to pick up some skin oil. Wipe the oil on your lips for short-term relief.

**Fight yeast with yogurt.** If the corners of your mouth appear red and cracked, you may have an overgrowth of yeast (a fungus), caused perhaps by antibiotics or stress. Go to the supermarket and pick up some yogurt containing live active cultures (check the label). Then, swish the yogurt around in your mouth several times a day. The live active cultures include *Lactobacillus acidophilus*, beneficial bacteria that control yeast.

**Cover up your kisser.** Always apply a lip balm with a sun protection factor (SPF) of 15 or higher before heading outside.

**Lick your problem, not your lips.** Licking your lips to moisturize them is only natural. Unfortunately, air evaporates the moisture, leaving your lips even drier than before.

provides some protection against sun damage. Combine these factors with exposure to blazing sun, strong winds, or moisture-sapping indoor heat, and you can understand why your lips sometimes become chapped.

## Cold Sores

Nothing can ruin a beautiful smile like a nasty-looking cold sore. And if you get one once, you're likely to get them again and again.

You can credit their persistence to herpes simplex type 1, the virus that causes cold sores. Ninety percent of the people who carry the virus picked it up during childhood. It lurks in your system forever, lying dormant among the nerve ganglia beneath your skin's surface, just waiting for something to activate it.

For women, that something is usually stress. When you're under stress, your resistance to disease drops. The virus seizes the opportunity to instigate an outbreak.

If you have ever had a cold sore before, you are probably familiar with what doctors call the prodrome—a sort of introductory itching around the area where a sore is about to erupt.

A cold sore usually sticks around for one to two weeks. You can use these natural remedies to minimize any discomfort and shorten the duration of an outbreak.

**Give it the cold shoulder.** The minute you feel a cold sore coming on, wrap an ice cube in a handkerchief and hold it directly on the sore for about five minutes. Repeat every two to three hours. No virus, including herpes simplex type 1, can survive in a cold environment.

**Try a little tenderizer.** Mix meat tenderizer with a few drops of water to make a paste. Apply the paste to the cold sore and hold it in place with a dry washcloth for 5 to 10 minutes. Repeat every two to three hours for the first day of an outbreak, then cut back the treatments to three times a day. Continue until the sore heals.

**Line up lysine.** Before the advent of the prescription drug acyclovir (Zovirax) for cold sores, people swore by the preventive and healing properties of lysine. This amino acid counteracts arginine, a substance in various foods that seems to trigger cold sores in some people. Lysine tablets are available in drugstores and health food stores.

**Shrink the sore with zinc.** An essential trace mineral, zinc is essential for proper wound healing—especially cell production—and helps get rid of cold sores more quickly. During an outbreak, take 30 milligrams of zinc a day with food or water. Once the sore heals, cut back to 15 milligrams a day.

*Note:* If you're taking more than 20 milligrams daily, it's a good idea to inform your doctor.

**Dab on some sun protection.** If you have had a cold sore in the past, wearing lip balm with an SPF of 30 at all times can help prevent another outbreak. You can find lip balms with high SPFs in sporting goods stores and drugstores. (During an outbreak, use a cotton swab to apply the balm to your lips and the outside border of the cold sore. That way, you won't transfer the virus to the balm stick.)

**Leave it alone.** If you have a cold sore, don't pull it, stretch it, or otherwise touch it. You could get very painful cold sores on your hand, especially if the fluid from the blister gets under a hangnail.

# Relief for Sore Eyes

Of all six senses, we rely on vision the most. In fact, a full 80 percent of the information that we gather from the world around us passes through our eyes.

With that kind of activity, our eyes are entitled to get a little tired and sore from time to time. But these days, eye problems seem more prevalent than ever. That's because we're devoting more time to what optometrists call near-point tasks—things such as gazing at computer and TV screens and reading the tiny type in stock reports and on food labels. Unfortunately, human eyes weren't designed for this kind of up-close work.

"Most common eye conditions—including bloodshot eyes and eyestrain—can have a functional cause, meaning that they occur because of the way we use our eyes," explains Anne Barber, O.D., director of program services for the Optometric Extension Program Foundation, an organization based in Santa Ana, California, that promotes vision education. "They're characteristic of a visual system that isn't functioning as efficiently as it should."

Regular exams are your best eye insurance because they'll catch any vision changes—as well as serious conditions such as cataracts, glaucoma, and macular degeneration—early on. Dr. Barber suggests that you see an optometrist or ophthalmologist every two years until you reach age 55, then every year thereafter. "If we catch a problem early on and start treating it right away, we stand a better chance of saving vision. So be sure your vision care provider does a full series of near-point vision tests and provides vision therapy to take care of functional problems or refers you to an office that does," she says.

For more run-of-the-mill eye conditions, proper self-care is usually sufficient. Eye doctors share these favorite natural remedies for keeping the eyes and eye area healthy.

## Bloodshot Eyes

As eye problems go, bloodshot eyes are easy to self-diagnose. You just have to look in the mirror. To bring those blood vessels down to size and get rid of the redness, follow this advice.

**Clear your eyes with cold.** Wrap ice cubes in a clean washcloth and lay the compress over your eyes for 30 minutes.

**Buy tears in a bottle.** Artificial tears ease the sting of bloodshot eyes and clear up the irritation that made you see red in the first place. You'll find these products in drugstores. (If you wear contacts, rewetting drops will work just as well.)

**Dispense with the medicated eyedrops.** Funny thing about over-the-counter medicated eyedrops such as Visine or Murine: The more you use them, the more you need them. It's a condition that doctors call rebound hyperemia. So reserve medicated eyedrops for occasional use.

## Crow's-Feet

The first signs of crow's-feet usually appear when we reach our late twenties. At that point, the tiny lines are visible only when we squint. They gradually deepen over the years and become prominent once we reach our forties.

The sooner you take steps to prevent crow's-feet, the younger the skin around your eyes will remain. But even if you already have lines, you can minimize their appearance.

**Fade lines with AHAs.** Alpha hydroxy acids (AHAs)—natural acids derived from foods such as fruits, sugarcane, and sour milk—diminish crow's-feet by sloughing off old skin cells and exposing younger cells underneath. AHAs also plump the skin and restore its ability to retain moisture. Look for an eye cream containing 5 percent AHAs. (Be careful to avoid your eyelids when applying.)

## EYEDROPS MADE EASY

The tough thing about putting in eyedrops is that you can't see what you're doing. More drops end up running down your face in the opposite direction!

Here's the no-fuss, no-drip way to self-administer eyedrops, from Anne Sumers, M.D., an ophthalmologist in Ridgewood, New Jersey, and spokesperson for the American Academy of Ophthalmology.

**Tilt your head back or lie down on the couch. Pull your lower lid away from your eye so that it forms a little pocket. Then, squeeze the eyedrop into the pocket. Do not let the dropper touch your eye or eyelid. Bacteria can contaminate the eyedropper if it touches you. Contact with the dropper can also scratch your cornea.**

Do the second eye immediately after the first. Then, after the drops are in, close your eyes for a minute or two and press your index fingers next to the corners of your eyes where they meet your nose. Keeping your eyes open or blinking will send the drops into the drainage duct between your eye and nose. If that happens, your eye won't benefit from the drops at all. In fact, if you're using a type of prescription drops called beta-blockers and it goes down into that duct, you could experience a slow or irregular heartbeat, says Dr. Sumers. But closing your eyes and pressing against them with your index fingers closes that duct so that drops stay in the eye where they belong.

Before opening your eyes, wipe away any lingering moisture from your closed lids. Finally, if you don't think the drop got into your eye, do it again. You can't overdose on eyedrops, says Dr. Sumers.

**Switch from alpha to beta.** If you have sensitive skin, use a product containing beta hydroxy acids. They reduce fine lines and wrinkles just as well as AHAs but with less irritation.

**Invest in cool shades.** Always wear wraparound sunglasses in bright or hazy outdoor light. Sunglasses may help prevent crow's-feet by stopping you from squinting.

**Stop rubbing your eyes.** The skin around your eyes can stretch and wrinkle in response to repeated rubbing.

## Dark Circles

Go ahead and blame Mom or Dad for those dark circles under your eyes. Contrary to popular belief, heredity— not lack of sleep—typically paints that bluish black or brownish tinge on the skin. While fatigue doesn't cause dark circles, it can certainly make them more pronounced. So can excessive sun exposure, as the sun's rays break down collagen and elastin. Allergies, illness, menstruation, and even pregnancy can also aggravate existing dark circles.

Medically speaking, dark circles under the eyes are harmless. Still, if you have them, you probably wish they were a little less noticeable. They can be, if you follow this advice.

**Count on chamomile.** Chamomile helps minimize dark circles by constricting the blood vessels, including those under the eyes. Place a steeped, chilled chamomile tea bag under each closed eye for 10 to 20 minutes in the morning, while you're waiting for the coffee to brew.

*Note:* Some pollen-sensitive people may be allergic to chamomile tea. Discontinue use if you experience any negative reaction.

**Let witch hazel do the work.** As an alternative to chamomile, soak cotton balls in witch

---

### REAL-LIFE SCENARIO
#### She's "Contacted" an Eye Problem

When Marie moved to Tucson, Arizona, last year to get relief from her allergies, she decided it was time for a total makeover. She took up exercise, got a new hairdo, started wearing makeup, and traded in her glasses (which she had been wearing since she was five) for contact lenses. At 35, she never looked better in her life, but she's having problems with her contact lenses. Even though she switched to makeup formulated for sensitive eyes, her eyes feel itchy and dry by the end of the day. She doesn't want to go back to wearing glasses but is worried that the contacts will ruin her eyes.

The reasons why Marie is having problems with her eyes are multiple, but they're not too big to overcome.

To begin with, most women's eyes tend to dry a bit after age 35, which is complicated even more by living in a dry climate such as Tucson. And if she takes antihistamines to control her allergies, they can make a dry problem even drier. Plus, eyes can be sensitive to makeup. So it's no wonder that her contacts are irritating her eyes. This doesn't mean, though, that she must go back to wearing glasses.

First, she should talk to her ophthalmologist about

---

hazel and lay them on the skin under your closed eyes for 20 minutes.

**Keep them hidden.** To cover dark circles, use a yellow-based stick concealer. Yellow neutralizes pink, red, and purple hues in the skin.

## Eye Irritations

Unless you wear protective goggles 24 hours a day, you're eventually going to get something in your eye. It could be a speck of dust, grit, or makeup. The longer it stays put, the more red, scratchy, and swollen your eye will become.

But foreign objects aren't the only things that irritate eyes. Smoke, pollen, and chlorine (in switching to a lens with a lower water content to prevent her eyes from dehydrating. She can also try over-the-counter moisturizing eyedrops, or artificial tears, which are especially helpful at the end of the day. And since she lives in a sunny climate, she should always wear sunglasses when outside. Sun is irritating on the eyes, too.

At home, Marie can create a more humid environment for her eyes by using air-conditioning less, running a humidifier, and keeping plants in the bedroom. Most important, she should give her eyes a rest and take her contacts out when she's in for the night. When she cleans her lenses, Marie should use a preservative-free solution, as preservatives can irritate sensitive eyes.

Marie's makeup may be adding to her problem, but it's probably not the main cause of her itchy eyes. Her eyelids would be itchy, red, and uncomfortable all day long if that were the case. But using a good makeup remover for sensitive eyes—baby shampoo is a good one—is still wise. The key, of course, is to get it all off.

**Expert consulted**
Anne Sumers, M.D.
Ophthalmologist
Ridgewood, New Jersey
Spokesperson for the American Academy
    of Ophthalmology

eye, remove it with the corner of a moist tissue.

**Let the water flow.** Ordinary tap water can flush a foreign object from your eye. Go to the sink, lean down close to the faucet, and splash water into your eye.

**Be bold with cold.** For irritation caused by an allergy, lay a washcloth soaked in fresh cold water over your eyes for 5 to 10 minutes.

**Make a shampoo solution.** Eye irritation sometimes results from blepharitis, a condition in which the eyelid margin (the thin edge of skin between your eyeball and eyelashes) becomes swollen from excess oil production. To treat blepharitis, add two or three drops of no-tears baby shampoo to one-third cup of water, dip a cotton swab into the solution, and run the swab along the bottom eyelid margin while your eye is open. Then close your eye and run the swab over the top eyelid margin where the lid meets the eyelashes. Use this remedy once or twice a day.

## Pinkeye

Feel as though a mosquito is permanently lodged underneath your eyelid? Are the whites of your eyes so irritated that they've turned pink or bloodshot red? Odds are that you have pinkeye.

Typically, pinkeye results from an allergy to pollen, pet dander, or certain chemicals or from a bacterial or viral infection. In fact, the same viruses that cause the common cold can also cause pinkeye. And like the common cold, infectious pinkeye is extremely contagious and easily spread by hand-to-eye contact.

Bacterial pinkeye is the most serious type, and unless it's treated with prescription medication, it can lead to loss of vision.

swimming pools) do the job just as well. If you have removed an irritant yet you have discharge coming from your eye or other abnormal symptoms, see your ophthalmologist. Irritation can also arise from a bacterial or viral infection.

Whatever its cause, eye irritation can usually be treated at home with simple self-care techniques. Here's what to do.

**Flip your lid.** If something is in your eye, you can use your eyelids to gently push the particle down and out. Grasp the eyelashes of your upper lid between your fingers, then pull the upper lid over the lower lid. This allows the lower lashes to brush the speck off the inside of your upper lid. If the particle moves to the corner of your

## FOLK REMEDY: DOES IT WORK?

### Cucumber Slices on Puffy Eyes

The old saying "cool as a cucumber" is probably what sparked the idea that putting cucumbers on your eyes can help reduce puffiness (much like an ice pack can reduce swelling).

"Puffy eyes are induced by things like crying, menstruation, or any other factor that may cause the body to retain fluid," says Mary Ruth Buchness, M.D., chief of dermatology at St. Vincent's Hospital and Medical Center in New York City. So even something as cool as a cucumber isn't going to take the fluid away.

The problem is that cucumbers may even make your eyes feel worse. They contain a substance that can cause an immediate reaction in the form of hives in some women.

**RECOMMENDATION: Forget It**

---

**Check out chickweed.** The herb chickweed helps fight infection, yet it's mild enough to use on your eyes. Brew a pot of chickweed tea and let it cool until it is comfortable to the touch. Then dip a clean cloth into the tea and hold the cloth against the affected eye while it's closed. Continue rewetting and reapplying the cloth for up to an hour.

**Get goldenseal.** If you have bacterial pinkeye, an eye bath of goldenseal tea can soothe your eyes and fight the infection. To make the eye bath, put one teaspoon of dried goldenseal into one cup of freshly boiled water. Steep for 10 minutes, then strain the mixture and allow the liquid to cool. Use an eyedropper to squirt two drops of the liquid into the affected eye.

**Leave your eyes *au naturel*.** Avoid wearing eye makeup while you have infectious pinkeye. Replace your mascara and liner. If your mascara wand or liner becomes contaminated, you'll just keep transferring the virus or bacteria from one eye to the other.

Seeing a doctor at the first sign of pinkeye is important. She can decide whether you require a prescription or you can manage the condition with self-care alone. Then use these strategies to help relieve the immediate symptoms and prevent the spread of germs.

**Remove your contacts.** If you wear contacts, take them out at the first sign of redness and irritation. Otherwise, they'll only exacerbate your discomfort and, if you have infectious pinkeye, they'll trap the germs in your eyes.

**Run hot and cold.** Alternating hot and cold compresses stimulates circulation and draws infection-fighting white blood cells to your eyes. Soak a clean washcloth in very warm water, wring it out, and hold it against your eyes for a minute. Then soak the cloth in cold water, wring it out, and hold it against your eyes for a minute. Repeat this process two or three times.

## Sties

Each of your eyelids contains eyelash follicles. Sometimes one of these follicles becomes infected, perhaps because it's clogged with dandrufflike scales or you have used a germ-laden mascara brush. Eventually, a painful red lump with a white head of pus sprouts at the base of the eyelash. This is what's known as a sty.

If you have a persistent or recurrent sty, see your doctor. It could be a sign of diabetes or a cyst. Also see a doctor if your sty doesn't get better or gets worse after two days.

As with a pimple on your face, a sty should

never be popped. It may rupture beneath the surface of the skin, aggravating the inflammation. Instead, heed this advice.

**Hold a hot potato.** Wrap a warm, damp washcloth around a hot baked potato (the cloth will retain the heat longer). Then hold the cloth against the affected, closed eye for five minutes. Repeat four times every day for two weeks. This will gently coax the sty to break open and heal.

**Give your eyes a break.** Stop wearing eye makeup until the sty heals. This means all eye makeup—mascara, eyeliner, and shadow. Otherwise, you may end up with several sties.

## Tired Eyes

Tired eyes, while uncomfortable, are seldom cause for alarm. Still, if your discomfort persists, you should see an ophthalmologist. You may need eyeglasses when you do close work.

To perk up tired eyes, try these tips.

**Look around.** The moment your eyes begin to bother you, look up from your work and into the distance. This lets your eye muscles relax.

**Put your palms to work.** Rub your hands together to warm them up a bit. Then gently position your palms over your closed eyes. Hold for five minutes, breathing easily while you do. This should rest and rejuvenate your eyes quite nicely.

**Squeeze out fatigue.** Take a deep breath while raising your shoulders and squeezing your eyes and fists as tightly closed as you can. Then exhale and relax all of the muscles at once. By tightening and releasing the voluntary muscles in your shoulders and fists, you can trick the involuntary muscles in your eyes into releasing as well.

## Under-Eye Bags

Women and women doctors alike often talk about baggy eyes and puffy eyes interchangeably. But there is a difference between the two.

Baggy eyes develop with age. As you grow older, the muscles under your eyes weaken, and the skin becomes less elastic. Fat tissue pushes through and around the muscles, giving the skin a swollen appearance. Once bags develop, you can't do much about them other than concealing them with makeup or having cosmetic surgery.

Puffy eyes, on the other hand, are temporary. They occur when something prompts your body to collect and retain fluid under the eyes. That something could be almost anything, including crying, lack of sleep, allergies, menstruation, or eating salty foods. If you awaken and find one eye swollen three times greater than the other, call your physician. This could be a sign of an allergic reaction to an insect bite, or hives. In addition, visit your doctor if your eyes don't close all the way (it could indicate thyroid disease).

As with baggy eyes, you can use makeup to mask puffy eyes. But to get rid of the puffiness for good, try these strategies.

**Spoon on relief.** One of the fastest, easiest, and cheapest ways to reduce puffiness around your eyes is with a glass of ice water and four metal serving spoons. Chill the spoons in ice water, then place one over each eye. When the spoons become warm, switch them with the others chilling in the glass of water.

**Make tea bag compresses.** Tea contains tannins, natural astringents that pull skin taut and reduce puffiness. Wrap two steeped tea bags that have cooled in tissue (so they won't stain your skin), then lay the bags over your closed eyes for two to five minutes.

**Dry out with dandelion.** A natural diuretic, the dandelion herb helps your body eliminate excess fluid. Drink a cup of dandelion leaf tea or take one-half teaspoon of dandelion leaf tincture three times a day. You can buy herbal tinctures, dried herbs, or teas in health food stores.

*Note:* Women who are taking diuretics, such as for high blood pressure, should not drink dandelion tea. And if you have gallbladder disease, do not use without your doctor's okay.

# Super Nail Solutions

The computer revolution has had at least one unexpected and as yet unexplained health benefit for women. All that tap-tap-tapping on computer keyboards appears to make fingernails grow faster and stronger.

Even if you're not computer-crazed, any activity that has you striking your nails against a hard surface—from playing the piano to drumming your fingers—can stimulate growth, according to Diana Bihova, M.D., a dermatologist in New York City and author of *Beauty from the Inside Out*. So can menstruation and pregnancy. "Weather is a factor, too," she says. "We don't exactly know why, but fingernails grow faster in summer."

## Hard As Nails

Of course, moving to warmer climes isn't the most practical way to get longer, stronger nails. Thankfully, you have more sensible options. The following strategies can keep your nails looking their best.

**Trim after you bathe.** Cutting your nails while they're dry leaves them vulnerable to damage. Instead, plan your manicure for after your bath or shower, when your nails are soft.

**Avoid cutting corners.** When trimming your nails, leave them square at the corners. This maximizes nail strength.

**File away flaws.** Keep an emery board in your purse or desk drawer. At the first sign of a nick or chip, use the board to smooth out the unevenness and prevent further damage. Always file in the same direction.

**Slather on moisturizer.** Apply moisturizer to your hands every time you wash them. Take a moment to massage the lotion into your skin and nails.

**Be prudent with polish remover.** Frequent use of nail polish remover can dry out your nails. So use remover sparingly, preferably no more than once a week. Look for an acetone-free product, which is less drying. Apply a small amount to a cotton ball, press it against the nail for about two seconds, then gently rub off the polish.

**Protect your mitts.** Whenever you wash dishes or use household cleaners, wear protective latex gloves with separate thin cotton gloves underneath. The cotton gloves help absorb perspiration. That's important because sweat makes hands soggy, further weakening nails.

## Brittle Nails

It's doubtful that any woman will get through life without getting brittle nails. Some of us are born with them. Others get them after years of submerging their hands in water or harsh household detergents. Getting older takes a toll, too: Almost everyone's nails become thinner with age.

So what can you do to restore moisture to your nails and keep them healthy and strong? For starters, try these tips.

**Offer 'em olive oil.** Immerse your fingertips in one-half cup of warmed olive oil and soak for 15 to 30 minutes.

**Break open the bath beads.** As an alternative to olive oil, break open three or four bath-oil capsules and empty their contents into one-half cup of warm water. Soak your fingertips in the diluted bath oil for five minutes.

**Make bedtime a formal affair.** Before going to bed, coat your nails and hands with a thick layer of petroleum jelly. Then slip on a pair of white cotton gloves to protect your hands overnight. You'll love the way this treatment makes your nails look.

**Go for a quick fix.** To salvage a split or broken nail, apply a very small amount of nail glue to the tear.

---

### A MANICURE FOR HEALTHY NAILS

Some manicures—French manicures or sculpted nails, for example—are designed to make your nails look great. Others are designed to make your nails look great and healthy. Here's the best way to buff and shine your nails to perfect health, according to Ida Orengo, M.D., associate professor of dermatology at Baylor College of Medicine in Houston.

 First, place your hands in a small dish of warm water mixed with mild detergent for five minutes to remove dirt and bacteria. "This will get your nails fresh and clean and avoid the possibility of pushing any bacteria under your cuticles while giving yourself a manicure," says Dr. Orengo. Dry your hands gently with a soft clean towel.

 While they're still soft, gently cut or clip your nails to about one-quarter inch in length. Hard, dry nails can crack or split when you cut them. One-quarter inch is the perfect length for strong nails. Anything longer can break, split, and chip more easily.

 With an orange stick wrapped in cotton, gently push back your cuticles. Cuticles should never be cut, says Dr. Orengo, because they protect your nails against bacterial and fungal infections.

 File your nails with an emery board. This also needs to be done while they're soft and pliable. Otherwise, they could split. File in one direction, from side to center, until they are squared off at the top. Filing in a back-and-forth motion can weaken and damage the nail, says Dr. Orengo. Filing nails to a point will also weaken your nails and cause them to break easily.

 Rub your nails with a nail moisturizing lotion. The lotion will hydrate your nails and prevent them from drying and cracking. "Rub the lotion liberally into your hands and nails," says Dr. Orengo. Wipe off the excess. Wait two or three minutes for the moisturizer to soak into your nails.

 Before applying color, brush on a clear pre-coat polish. The clear polish will prevent your nails from turning yellow.

 To prevent your nails from drying out, remove polish with a non-acetone remover no more than once a week, says Dr. Orengo.

Reinforce the tear by covering it with a small piece of tissue from a tea bag. Let the glue dry completely, then use a fine buffer to even out the nail surface. (Be sure to leave the tissue in place.) Finally, apply a top coat over the tissue.

## Hangnails

A hangnail forms when a small piece of skin tears away from your finger right by the nail bed. Even though it's tiny, it can be quite painful and even bleed.

If you get a hangnail, don't pick at it or try to bite it off. It can actually become infected. To re-move a hangnail the right way, use this three-step technique.

**Start by softening.** Never cut off a hangnail while it's dry. Instead, soften it by soaking it in warm water and olive oil.

**Clip it cleanly.** Use nail scissors or nail clippers to remove the hangnail. Cut it as short as you can without damaging the skin around it.

**Apply the finishing touches.** After clipping the hangnail, massage the skin around your nail with moisturizer, cover it with an adhesive bandage, and leave it alone.

## Sore Cuticles

That tiny rim of near-transparent tissue at the base of each nail is there for a reason. It serves as a barrier, protecting the nail against infection.

To repair damaged cuticles and keep them problem-free, add these steps to your nail-care routine.

**First, soak them.** Before you do anything to your cuticles, soften them in warm sudsy water for several minutes. This prevents drying and cracking.

**Then give them a gentle push.** Wrap the tip of an orange stick in cotton gauze. Then use the stick to gently push back each cuticle.

**Finish with petroleum jelly.** After pushing back your cuticles, massage them with a thin layer of petroleum jelly to seal in moisture.

# PART THREE

# Our
# Bodies

# Banish the Monthly Blues

If there's anything that we can depend on to be undependable, it's our periods. They may arrive like clockwork each month, but how they're going to act is anyone's guess. Menstrual symptoms seem to have minds of their own.

To deal with these constant yet ever-changing facts of life, many women turn to old standbys such as ibuprofen and over-the-counter diuretics. While usually good for pain and water retention, these medications don't treat all the symptoms that bother women—and they can have unwanted side effects, says Jennifer Brett, N.D., a naturopathic physician in Stratford, Connecticut. "They don't deal with the underlying cause of the problems, either," she says.

Many natural remedies, including herbs, diet, and yoga, can help. While Mother Nature's treatments might seem new to you, women actually used them long before the advent of ibuprofen. "It is only recently that we've turned to pills to make us feel better," Dr. Brett says.

Natural relief for the monthly blues involves more than taking something to alleviate symptoms. Healthy lifestyle changes such as eating right and exercising can prevent problems that come with your period, Dr. Brett says. For natural solutions to monthly problems, try the following.

## Cramps

For almost half of us, our periods announce their arrival with some kind of pain. It can last for as little as an hour or as long as three days. Why does it put on such a show?

When hormones called prostaglandins are released during your period, the uterine blood vessels constrict and decrease blood flow to the area. As a result, the uterine muscle clenches tightly, and you feel it as a cramp.

Many of the world's traditional, natural healing systems treat cramps successfully.

**Calm cramps with herbs.** Black haw and cramp bark both have a long history of use to relax the muscles of the uterus. If your cramps are mild, make a tea: Add two teaspoons of dried black haw or cramp bark per cup of water. Boil for 10 minutes, cool, and strain; drink up to three cups a day.

Severe cramps may require stronger medicine.

Try a teaspoon of black haw or cramp bark tincture (sometimes labeled as an herbal extract) every half-hour for two to three hours. It is best not to wait until your pain peaks to start dosing.

If you are routinely plagued with cramps, you should start taking the herbs a few days before you expect your period. Since these herbs, which can be purchased at health food stores, contain an aspirin-like compound, do not use them if you are sensitive to aspirin. Don't take black haw if you have a history of kidney stones.

**Heat things up.** The soothing effect of lying in a tub of hot water helps relax tense uterine muscles, therefore easing your cramps.

Or you can make your own heating pad. Dampen a terry-cloth towel in comfortably hot water. Wring it out and test it for temperature before placing it over your crampy lower abdomen. Then relax and let the towel cool naturally.

**Relieve pressure with pressure.** Press the traditional Chinese acupressure points for relieving menstrual cramps. These points are located at the groin, in the middle of the crease where each of your legs joins your trunk. You can press there with your fingertips, or you can stimulate both points at once by positioning your left fist over the points on your left side and your right fist on the right side. Then, lying on your stomach with your fists in·place, use the weight of your body to apply pressure to the areas for at least two minutes.

**Acupressure Points**

**Pour a glass of water.** Here's another use of water to relieve menstrual cramps—drink it! No one is sure why it works, but scientific research shows that increased hydration relieves menstrual cramps. If you have cramps, drink as much water as you can until the cramps go away.

**Stretch out.** Your lower back and thighs may ache when cramps stimulate nerves that supply these areas. Stretching yoga-style can help.

Sit on the floor with your legs together and stretched in front of you, your arms by your sides with your hands touching the floor. Bend your right leg out to the side and bring your foot next to your left inner thigh.

Inhale. Push into the floor with your hands to lift your chest and lengthen your spine upward; twist your torso to the left so that your breastbone is directly over your extended leg. As you exhale, bend forward from the hips, keeping your back straight. Reach forward and grasp your left foot with both hands (use a belt instead of your hands if necessary). Do not hunch your spine. Stay stretched for two to three minutes.

**Give yourself a rubdown.** For quick relief, add five drops each of warming, muscle-relaxing essential oils of wintergreen and lavender to a one-half-ounce base of olive or almond oil. Rub it over your abdomen or lower back, then apply a heating pad—for no more than 20 minutes at a time—covered by a thin towel and set on low.

## Endometriosis Pain

As disorders go, endometriosis is as mysterious as it sounds. Normally, the endometrial tissue—the soft, blood-rich lining of your uterus—thickens and is shed each month. But in some women, endometrial tissue migrates outside the uterus and starts to grow on and around other pelvic organs, such as the ovaries, colon, and bladder, or the fallopian tubes.

The renegade tissue may exert pressure on the

## AUNT EMMA HAS ARRIVED!

From "Aunt Flo" to "falling off the roof" and beyond, women's monthly menstrual periods have earned many nicknames. These euphemisms evolved as a secret language, code words that girls and women used for privacy when boys and men were around. Here are just a few.

Menstruation has been called "the curse" inflicted on all women—thanks to Eve and her sins in the Garden of Eden, according to one notion. Perhaps due to cramps and inconvenience, this natural event has also been dubbed "a package of troubles." There's the colorful trip down "red road." And for those who prefer a crude medical description for "that time of the month" consider the term "falling off the roof," which refers to the fact that a woman's menstrual flow seems to be falling from a high place, like the top (or roof) of her womb.

It can be an "old friend" or an unwanted (or in some instances, wanted) "visitor." Sometimes this visitor has a name, such as "Bloody Mary." Or it's a relative, such as "Aunt Emma from Reading" or "my country cousin." Menstruation has also been referred to as just a familiar pal: "my red-headed friend from the South."

Some women have described their periods in terms of their preferred sanitary product. If you use tampons, your "plug is in" or it's a "white cylinder week." Wear sanitary napkins? You may be riding "the white pony." (Of course, the mere mention that you are "on the rag" warns friends that you may be a bit moody.)

Around your mate, the nickname of choice may reflect your sexual availability. You may issue a warning: "red alert," "my red flag is up," or "I'm flying baker" (a reference to the navy signal that means "keep off").

---

cycle of pain, stress, and more pain. Close your eyes, take a few deep breaths, and tense the muscles in your face. Hold for a few seconds, then take a deep breath and release. Repeat this for your neck, shoulders, arms, and on down through your body.

Since progressive relaxation needs to be practiced, do it regularly, not just when the pain is bad.

**Increase your bioflavonoids.** Bioflavonoids seem to reduce excessive bleeding by strengthening capillary walls. These vitamin C–related substances, found in citrus fruit, garlic, onions, and all other vegetables, may also help lower excessively high estrogen levels. So eat your fruit and veggies and take 1,000 milligrams of bioflavonoids daily as a supplement. Look for these supplements at health food stores.

**Cut down on animal fat.** Eat less meat, fatty fish and poultry, dairy products, and eggs, and you may reduce your exposure to dioxins, which are chemical residues that may be linked to both the onset and severity of endometriosis.

**Buy pads or unbleached tampons.** Avoid regular tampons, which owe their pure white appearance to a bleaching process that leaves dioxins behind in the cotton. Switch to sanitary pads or look for 100 percent unbleached, organic cotton tampons.

organs and result in pain. Endometriosis may also lead to painful sex, infertility, or both.

Endometriosis can't be cured, but you can control the pain and possibly the growth of the tissue by natural means. Here's how.

**Practice relaxation.** By systematically tensing and relaxing individual muscle groups in your body, you can release tension and slow the

## Heavy Bleeding

An occasional change in your monthly flow is perfectly normal and may be due to a lifestyle change. Have you started a new exercise program? Taken a new job? Moved into a new home?

Age could also be a factor: Your uterus keeps growing until you're around age 35, so there's more uterine lining to bleed. Approaching menopause can also bring unpredictable, heavy periods. You should pay attention to your cycle so you know what's normal for you, and be certain to have an annual examination.

If bleeding or pain seems unusually severe for you or if you miss a period, see a doctor. If she rules out possible underlying medical causes for heavy bleeding, these suggestions may ease the problem.

**Eat iron-rich foods.** Inadequate iron intake may cause excessive bleeding. The most efficiently absorbed iron is supplied by foods such as red meat, liver, egg yolks, and fish.

If you're watching your fat intake, a multivitamin/mineral supplement with iron is a sound alternative. Vegetarians can get iron from grains, beans, and dried fruit, but they must also take vitamin C to enhance absorption.

**Reach for a raspberry infusion.** According to herbal medical lore, a cup a day of raspberry leaf infusion acts as a tonic for the ovaries and uterus. To make it, add about four tablespoons of dried raspberry leaves to a quart of boiling water, then remove it from the heat and let it stand overnight.

**Mix a bark and valerian cocktail.** Heavy bleeding accompanied by nasty cramps responds well to a blend of three teaspoons cramp bark tincture mixed with five teaspoons valerian tincture. Take between 40 drops and one teaspoon of this blend in small amounts of warm water up to three times a day if necessary. Since every

## WOMEN ASK WHY

**Why don't we ever hear about toxic shock syndrome anymore?**

Toxic shock syndrome (TSS), a rare but potentially deadly disease associated with tampon use, just isn't as prevalent as it used to be, thanks to new awareness among women who use tampons and perhaps to new standards for tampon absorbency.

While TSS doesn't make the news as often these days, it still affects up to 17 out of every 100,000 menstruating women and girls each year. Experts suspect that this illness is caused by bacteria entering the bloodstream, and it has been linked to the use of high-absorbency tampons. (Tampons seem to create an ideal breeding ground for bacteria.) Some research has shown that 8 out of 10 cases of TSS were among women who used this type of tampon.

You can avoid TSS by choosing the tampon with the minimum absorbency needed to manage your menstrual flow and by changing tampons frequently. Never go more than eight hours without switching to a fresh one. And don't wear tampons exclusively. Alternating tampons with pads can reduce the risk of TSS. If you experience any warning signs of TSS—sudden fever, vomiting, diarrhea, fainting or dizziness, or a rash that looks like sunburn—remove the tampon immediately and call your doctor.

*Expert consulted*
*Mary Beth Hasselquist, M.D.*
*Staff physician*
*Group Health Cooperative of Puget Sound*
*Clinical assistant professor*
*University of Washington*
*Seattle*

woman's cramps are different, the dose that works will be unique as well.

## Mood Swings

Women report more mood swings—more dips into depression and free falls into anxiety—

than men. The hormonal changes that women undergo before menstruation may make us more susceptible to downward spins. Even when you're feeling most vulnerable, though, you can lessen the severity of mood swings and even head some off at the pass. Here's how.

**Take a deep breath.** Ease emotional upheaval by practicing deep breathing for 5 to 10 minutes at least twice a day. Deep breathing helps the nervous system and endocrine system to balance and calm down, easing the emotional ups and downs associated with premenstrual syndrome (PMS).

Sit up straight or lie on your back. Exhale through your nose, then inhale through your nose, focusing on your breath. Make exhalations and inhalations of equal lengths.

**Take action now.** If you feel yourself slipping into depression or anxiety, get up and do something—take a walk or clean the clutter off your desk. It doesn't matter what it is, as long as you engage in some type of physical activity.

**Get to bed.** You're especially vulnerable to mood swings when you're sleep-deprived, so be sure to get enough shuteye, particularly when you know that swings are more probable.

## Premenstrual Syndrome

It's not all in your head. You really do want to hang a Do Not Disturb sign around your neck the week before your period. Your cravings for chocolate are utterly overwhelming. And your favorite pants just won't zip shut.

But you've resolved not to give in to premen-

## WOMAN TO WOMAN
### Her Symptoms Just Disappeared

*When she was in her midthirties, Bonita Cochrane, a teacher from Long Island, began having irregular periods—and things got worse from there. After years of sporadic symptoms, she consulted a naturopathic physician, who confirmed what she had always suspected—that she was going through the premenopausal period known as perimenopause. Natural treatments relieved her symptoms and turned her life around. Here's her story.*

My story begins at the age of 34, with the onset of irregular periods. At around 38, I gained 25 to 30 pounds seemingly overnight. I had always exercised and eaten right, but I couldn't shed the weight no matter what I did.

I also became extremely bloated and moody and had other PMS symptoms, which I'd never experienced before.

When I hit 41, these symptoms, which would usually come and go, got worse. I was also so hot that my body felt like a raging fire—in February!

I found a naturopath who listened to my complaints and then, there in the office, prepared a homeopathic medicine called Lachesis. This substance, which comes from the venom of a bushmaster snake, is used to treat a variety of female reproductive problems, including perimenopause and PMS. Within 15 minutes of taking it, I felt better. She also

strual discomfort. So what's a real woman, beset with the very real symptoms of PMS, to do?

**Eat a little—a lot.** Eating five small meals a day, with a good balance of complex carbohydrates and a moderate amount of protein, can ease food cravings and mood swings. Half a turkey sandwich on whole-wheat bread, half a whole-wheat bagel spread with low-fat or fat-free cream cheese, or a cup of chicken-vegetable soup with whole-wheat crackers are good examples.

**Drink a drop of chasteberry.** Take 5 to 15

gave me Lachesis pills to take at home. Within two weeks, I was a changed woman.

The story doesn't end there, though. Shortly before I turned 42, I experienced very, very heavy bleeding during my period. I went to my gynecologist, but I wasn't satisfied with what he had to say, so I went back to my naturopath. She added everything up—the heavy bleeding, continued bloating, overheating, and irritability. She suggested that I was going through perimenopause.

She gave me a prescription for a combination herbal product containing chasteberry, St.-John's-wort, Siberian ginseng, shepherd's purse, and mugwort. I took one dose. After a good night's sleep, I felt calm. The hurricane that had been spinning around inside me was quiet. It was remarkable. For six months, I took the herbs every day as directed by my naturopath. Now, because my symptoms have abated so dramatically, I take it only now and then.

Since then, I've added other natural treatments to control my perimenopausal symptoms. For example, I take natural progesterone in pill form for the last 13 days of my cycle. I also take a natural substance called Isocort for what my naturopath calls adrenal support. With the help of these natural treatments, my symptoms are under control. My periods have returned to normal, like they were when I was a teenager. The bloating is gone, and I've even dropped a few pounds.

It really is unbelievable. My life is my own again.

drops of chasteberry tincture, mixed with a few ounces of water, three times a day. Chasteberry, also called vitex, is commonly prescribed in Europe for PMS.

**Maximize your magnesium.** Magnesium plays an important part in the treatment of PMS, according to some studies. Taking 300 milligrams of magnesium every day is associated with fewer cramps, less water retention, and an overall improvement in premenstrual symptoms. You'll also find magnesium in nuts, legumes, whole grains, and green vegetables.

## Tender Breasts

For most women, breast discomfort waxes and wanes with their menstrual cycles. Right before and during menstruation, higher-than-usual levels of estrogen may cause one or both breasts to swell and become tender. Know your body and what to expect each month. Any unusual increase in pain or discomfort calls for a visit to your doctor.

For tender breasts, here's what to do.

**Comfort with a warm compress.** Holding a warm compress such as a heated towel or towel-wrapped heating pad against the breast for 10 to 15 minutes can give some relief.

**Ice the swelling.** For some women, the uncomfortable swelling of breast tissue that often occurs before and during a menstrual period can be relieved with cold compresses. Wrap ice packs in towels, mold them around your breasts, and keep them there until the packs warm. Repeat as needed.

**Keep your glass filled.** Drink at least eight eight-ounce glasses of water a day. Paradoxically, the more water you drink, the less likely it is that your breasts will swell before your period.

**Get enough fiber.** Consume at least 30 grams of fiber a day. Both kinds of fiber—soluble and insoluble—help escort excess estrogen from your body, which prevents the hormone from stimulating breast tissue and causing discomfort.

**Reduce your dietary fat.** Limit your intake of dietary fat to 15 percent of calories. In one study, women who adhered to this guideline reported significant reductions in breast tenderness, swelling, and lumpiness.

# Ease Childbirth and Recovery

If you worry about pain or discomfort during pregnancy or childbirth, take comfort in this lesson from human history: Millions of women through the ages have given birth to millions of healthy babies—successfully *and* naturally.

"In this country, we probably have a pretty high fear quotient compared to other cultures," says certified nurse-midwife Marion Mc-Cartney, director of professional services for the American College of Nurse-Midwives in Washington, D.C. "I was in practice for 24 years in the Washington area, and I've worked with a lot of pregnant women from other countries. They seem to look at pregnancy and childbirth simply as natural events that women are quite capable of performing."

Of course, this natural event isn't always a comfortable one. You may experience morning sickness, you will certainly have some labor pain, and after delivery, you may find yourself coping with episiotomy pain, postpartum depression, or the aftermath of a cesarean section.

Where can you turn for relief? Often, drugs are out of the question. Moms-to-be must avoid most prescription and over-the-counter medica-tions during pregnancy (unless advised otherwise by their doctors) in order to protect the growing fetus. After delivery, if you're breast-feeding, you'll want to keep your breast milk free of medicines.

Happily, drug-free doesn't mean remedy-free. The pains and troubles that accompany pregnancy and its aftermath can be soothed with natural techniques. Read on to discover a world of natural solutions for moms-to-be and new moms, too. To play it safe, however, don't take anything while pregnant or nursing without consulting with your doctor first.

## Morning Sickness

The nausea, vomiting, and misery known as morning sickness can leave you feeling that this baby thing just might be a bad idea. Don't worry, it won't last. For most women, morning sickness disappears by the end of the first trimester. And you could be one of the lucky ones: Only about half of all pregnant women experience it.

What's behind this queasiness? Experts say that during pregnancy, increased hormone activity slows down your digestion, which can cause nausea. Fortunately, natural medicine offers safe remedies. Here are some of the best.

**Take a gingerly approach.** Sip some soothing, spicy ginger tea. This herb has an age-old reputation for settling out-of-sorts stomachs. In one study, women with the worst form of morning sickness, hyperemesis gravidarum, who took 250 milligrams of powdered ginger four times a day had a significant reduction in the number of attacks.

The fresh herb contains more of the active ingredients than powdered ginger. Make an anti–morning sickness tea by chopping about a one-quarter-inch piece of fresh ginger into small cubes. Place them in a non-aluminum pot, add one cup of water, cover, and simmer for 15 to 20 minutes. Keep the pot covered so that you don't boil away the volatile oils that are the active ingredients in this herb. Let cool and slowly sip up to two to three cups daily.

**Sip some morning mint tea.** Spearmint tea, sipped first thing in the morning, is effective against nausea. To make an infusion, pour one quart boiling water over one ounce dried mint leaves in a quart glass canning jar. Cover tightly and let the mint leaves steep overnight or for at least four hours. Then refrigerate. If kept refrigerated, the tea will last for up to a week.

*Note:* Be sure to choose spearmint and not peppermint, which may be too strong for a growing fetus's nervous system.

## WOMEN ASK WHY

### Why do I get weird cravings when I'm pregnant?

Some cravings stem from real physical needs. Others (like the classic pickles and ice cream) may just reflect cultural expectations—since pregnant women are supposed to get crazy eating urges, we sometimes respond by actually having them.

But before you dismiss a craving, consider whether it might be helping you to have a healthy pregnancy. A sudden desire for milk, juice, vegetables, or protein foods may be a signal that your body needs more nutrients—or at least more calories—to support a growing baby.

Some intense cravings come from very specific needs. Women who have diabetes during pregnancy tend to crave liquids, for a perfectly sensible reason. Diabetes raises blood sugar levels, which prompts more frequent urination. The result? Thirst for more liquids to replace what's been lost.

Women with anemia, a condition that becomes more common during pregnancy, often make up for their iron deficiencies by craving more green leafy vegetables or other iron-rich foods like liver.

What eludes science, however, are the reasons for other unusual cravings common in pregnant women with anemia. Some anemic women crave ice and can't make ice cubes fast enough to satisfy their need. Others crave starch and wouldn't bat an eyelash at eating right out of a box of cornstarch.

As silly as a craving may seem to you, it might reflect an underlying nutritional need, so it's worth mentioning to your obstetrician or midwife at your next visit. And what if your nutritional status is healthy, yet you just can't stop thinking about, say, chocolate ice cream? Indulge moderately.

**Expert consulted**
Linda Bradley, M.D.
Department of gynecology
Cleveland Clinic Foundation
Cleveland

**Quaff (or sniff) some lemons.** The taste and scent of lemon seem to quash queasiness. Try lemonade or make lemon water by squeezing some fresh lemon into cool water.

**Make your point.** An acupressure point in your wrist can help relieve nausea. The point is on the underside of your forearm, about 1½ inches away from your wrist and dead center between the ligaments. Press it with the pad of your thumb and hold for a slow count of 10. Breathe normally and repeat until the nausea subsides.

**Head for the seas.** Developed for motion sickness and available at drugstores, Sea-Bands apply constant pressure to acupressure points for nausea. Or you can try a do-it-yourself-version: Affix a dried bean like a kidney bean over the point with an adhesive bandage and wear it overnight.

**Stay hydrated with watermelon.** If you can't keep juice or water down, eat a few chunks of ice-cold watermelon. The water content will help keep you hydrated, and pregnant women can usually tolerate it without getting sick.

## Labor Pain

It's not hard to figure out where it got its name. Birthing a baby is hard labor—literally. Natural remedies can help ease the pain and prepare your body for the work ahead so that you stay more comfortable.

**Drink raspberry tea.** Drink one to two cups of raspberry leaf tea each week during your second trimester, building up to one cup a day during your third trimester. Raspberry leaf is considered a tonic herb. It contains an abundance of minerals and other compounds that help tone the muscular layer of the uterus.

To make the tea, steep one teaspoon of dried herb in a cup of freshly boiled water for 10 to 15 minutes and strain. You can buy the herb in health food stores.

**Do Kegel exercises.** To strengthen and tone muscles used during childbirth, this routine works your pelvic-floor muscles, which support the pelvic organs. The key to performing Kegels correctly is squeezing the muscles as though you were trying to stop the flow of urine. Hold for a count of 10, then release. Do 20 repetitions five times a day. You can do them anywhere.

**Vary your positions.** Changing positions frequently during labor may distract you somewhat from the pain and may even relieve some discomfort.

**Press away pain.** Using your thumbs, apply pressure to the left and right sides of your sacrum (the triangular bone at the base of your spine). This acupressure technique works especially well if you are having back labor, in which pain settles into your lower back. You will know when you have hit the right points. They will feel tender at first, but as you press them, the pain will ease.

**Add some heat.** Warm compresses are really helpful. A warm washcloth placed on your lower abdomen right above your pubic bone, either during or between contractions, is fine.

**Take a shower.** When the pain gets intense, a warm shower can help. The warmth of the water provides comfort and relaxation and can make labor more tolerable.

## Episiotomy Pain

Sometimes, under the force of expelling a full-term baby, the tissues between the vulva and anus tear or the pelvic muscles weaken and lead to a bulge in the bladder or rectum. To prevent tearing in this tender area (called the perineum), physicians and midwives sometimes take preemptive action and make a neat, clean cut (an episiotomy) to enlarge the birth opening. The incision is stitched up after delivery.

You can take the following natural steps to encourage healing and reduce pain and swelling in this sensitive area. If the pain worsens or doesn't subside within two weeks or if you experience sudden bleeding, your incision may be infected. Call your doctor right away.

**Chill out the swelling.** To reduce inflammation, apply an ice pack to the incision as needed for 15 to 20 minutes at a time for the first 12 hours after delivery. Look for cold packs that are about the size of sanitary pads and contain dry ice; they're sold in drugstores and medical supply stores. Remember to wrap it in a towel to prevent skin damage.

**Take a sitz bath.** Relaxing in a tub of water, either a shallow sitz bath or a deep regular bath, provides relief.

One study compared cold sitz baths with warm ones. The researcher found that the women who took cold soaks had less pain afterward because cold acts as an analgesic.

**Wash with herbs.** To soothe tenderness, relieve inflammation, aid healing, protect against bacteria, and improve circulation, try this herbal combination. Put one handful each of calendula flowers, comfrey root, yarrow flowers, and rosemary leaves into a pint of boiling water. Remove from the heat, cover, and steep for several minutes. Strain the liquid and transfer it to a plastic squirt bottle.

When the liquid has cooled to room temperature, use it to wash your vaginal area after you urinate. Or you can make a large batch and use it in a sitz bath. Simply pour the room-temperature liquid into a clean, shallow pan large enough to sit in, then do exactly that—sit in it for 10 to 15 minutes. You can store the solution in the refrigerator for two to three days.

**Try vitamin E.** Vitamin E has skin-healing properties and is often prescribed to people who have undergone surgery. If you have had an episiotomy, wait a couple of weeks for the laceration

to heal a little—that is, when the incision is knitting back together, no longer weeps any fluid, and shows no signs of infection.

## Breastfeeding Problems

Breastfeeding is as natural as breathing, but nursing doesn't always come naturally for mother or child. A newborn doesn't always "get it" right away. Perhaps your body doesn't seem to produce enough milk to satisfy your child, or nursing leaves your breasts sore. Don't despair: Women doctors have plenty of helpful advice.

One warning, however: If nothing you try relieves the pain and discomfort brought on by nursing, consult your doctor, especially if your breasts become red, hot, swollen, and painful. You may have mastitis, a breast infection that requires attention.

**Relax in your rocking chair.** If your baby is fussy, take some time to relax. Babies can sense insecurity and tension in their moms. Colic in babies has been associated with maternal tension. Being stressed also interferes with letting down your milk—that is, its release by your milk-producing glands.

**Massage out the milk.** When your milk isn't flowing, a gentle breast massage can stimulate it. With your fingertips, circle around the base of one breast, then the other. Then place both hands flat on either side of one breast and slowly slide outward from the areola, the dark area surrounding the nipple.

**Add some warmth.** It's not unusual for a milk duct to clog, preventing free flow of milk. A warm washcloth or shower and some gentle massage helps unplug a clogged milk duct by increasing blood flow to the area.

**Deflate breast discomfort.** An ancient folk remedy works well for tender, engorged breasts during the first few days following delivery: Place cool, fresh cabbage leaves on your breasts

## PROBLEM-FREE BREASTFEEDING

Infants are born with the right reflexes and instincts to breastfeed. What comes naturally to babies, however, may not come so naturally to new moms. Here are steps you can take to ensure breastfeeding success, says Jane Anderson, M.D., associate clinical professor of pediatrics at the University of California in San Francisco.

Start by finding a comfortable place and position. Cradle your baby so that she is facing you. You can help her get the nipple securely in her mouth if you make it protrude by holding your breast just beneath the nipple with your first two fingers. Once your baby is suckling contentedly, you can cradle her with both arms.

**Hold your baby so that her entire body is facing your breasts. Rest her head in the crook of your elbow and support her bottom with one hand.**

Avoid using bottles or rubber nipples for the first three weeks. Your baby must use a different sucking action to get milk from a bottle, so alternating between rubber nipples and your breast can confuse her.

After you've been nursing for a while, you may experience painful, cracked nipples that make breastfeeding unpleasant. You can ease the pain by changing the baby's position and allowing your nipples to air-dry after nursing. If these tips don't relieve your discomfort, your baby may not be latching on correctly. Discuss it with your doctor.

until they wilt fully (the cabbage leaves, that is, not your breasts).

If you're fresh out of cabbage leaves or prefer a less exotic approach, a cool, moist washcloth may help. Applying a cold compress for 15 to 20 minutes at a time between feedings reduces blood flow and overfilling of the breasts. But don't apply a compress just before feeding, as it will interfere with letdown of your milk.

**Change positions.** Using a variety of positions encourages your baby's mouth to create pressure on different parts of your nipple, which helps to prevent soreness as well as clogged ducts.

**Soothe with lotion.** If your nipples become dry and cracked, try between-feeding applications of a form of purified lanolin such as Lansinoh, made especially for nursing mothers. Be sure to thoroughly wash off the lotion before the baby's next feeding, though.

## Postpartum Depression

It's sometimes called the baby blues—the emotional slump that, for reasons that are not well understood, new moms sometimes experience after their babies arrive.

Postpartum depression has been linked to the hormonal changes that occur after birth. The stress of adjusting to life with an utterly dependent and totally demanding new person—one who cries and keeps you up nights—can also be part of the cause. Your mood should lighten after a week or two, although some women suffer for months if they don't get help. If you're feeling blue, here's what you can do to help lift your spirits.

**Keep taking your prenatal vitamins.** Symptoms of depression can result from shortages of certain vitamins, including folic acid, $B_6$, and $B_{12}$. You can take supplements for up to three months after delivery or for as long as you breastfeed your baby.

**Try aromatherapy.** Try gently sniffing the essential oil extracted from *Pelargonium graveolens*, a species of geranium. It's available at most health food stores. The aroma affects the adrenal cortex, the part of your brain that's responsible for establishing hormonal balance.

**Take frequent naps.** Catch up on your sleep whenever you can. Sleep deprivation is a tried-and-true method of torturing prisoners. It can lead to exhaustion, irritability, and irrationality. Forget about the dirty dishes and the laundry and try to sleep whenever your baby naps.

## Recovering from a C-Section

If you have a baby by cesarean section, you'll face all of the typical challenges and joys of new motherhood, plus one: the need to gain strength and heal after major surgery.

Natural therapies after a C-section can help boost your body's

## WOMAN TO WOMAN
### *Creativity Got Her through C-Section*

*Melissa Werger-León, a 32-year-old attorney from New York, had her dreams of natural childbirth dashed when she learned that she had to have an emergency cesarean section. But a little creativity and imagery helped her overcome the disappointment and pain. Here's her story.*

I wanted to have my baby Isak naturally. I took childbirth preparation classes, sweated through maternal fitness workouts, and read dozens of books. My pregnancy was textbook perfect, and at every checkup, my doctors said everything was fine.

But Isak's due date came and went. The next two weeks came and went. At my last doctor's appointment, I was running out of amniotic fluid, and Isak's heart rate had dropped. I was rushed to the hospital. When they told me I was going to have an emergency C-section, I was intensely relieved.

The reality of the pain that follows a C-section hit later. The hospital put me on two different pain medications, but I wanted to keep away from drugs. Also, the self-administered morphine had me vomiting and hallucinating. So I stopped taking it, and after two very uncomfortable days, one of the nurses suggested that I drink ginger tea for the pain. After that, I drank double-strength, warm ginger tea and cold ginger ale all day, which really helped.

Then, when I got home with Isak five days later, super-reality hit. I realized that all the furniture in our house is very low and that it was too painful to bend down to reach anything to care for my baby. My husband worked fast to accommodate my new needs, raising shelves, rearranging furniture, and moving Isak's diapers to a higher location.

Then there was the problem of the toilet. But I remembered those elevated toilet seat risers—like plastic doughnuts that are inches higher than standard toilet seats. I got one and put it on the toilet, and it helped immensely.

Looking back now, I realize that it's hard to prepare for a C-section. It sounds scary. But I can honestly say, don't be scared—to have a baby is worth the pain and difficulty.

ability to knit together the layers of skin and muscle that were opened during the surgery. Herbal helpers can aid the healing process.

**Supplement with nutrients.** Women who have had C-sections might want to take zinc (15 to 30 milligrams), bioflavonoids (500 to 1,000 milligrams), vitamin C (1,000 to 3,000 milligrams), vitamin E (400 international units), and evening primrose oil as supplements for four to six weeks. They help tissue mend and reduce inflammation.

**Try homeopathic healing.** A post–C-section treatment plan can also include two homeopathic remedies. Take a single 1M dose of homeopathic Arnica within the first day after surgery, then take a 6C or 12C dose of Arnica twice daily for a week after that. In addition, on the second day after surgery, take a 200C dose of Staphisagria. Both are believed to prevent some swelling and tenderness. Do not ingest nonhomeopathic arnica. (Homeopathic remedies can be found in health food stores.)

**Combine comfrey and calendula.** Once your incision begins to heal, you can help support the healing process with a skin wash made with comfrey and calendula. Calendula contains substances that reduce inflammation, combat infection, and even help the skin mend itself. Research shows that comfrey contains allantoin, a substance that prompts tissue repair, plus rosmarinic acid, which reduces swelling.

Combine equal parts of the two herbs, then make the wash by steeping one tablespoon of the mixture in two cups of freshly boiled water for 10 to 15 minutes. Let cool to room temperature. Twice a day, gently pour some of the mixture onto the incision and let it stay—don't rinse. You can also use sterile gauze pads or a clean washcloth to apply the wash. The wash can be stored in the refrigerator for up to three days.

Comfrey can heal the skin surface so quickly that it seals over unhealed tissue beneath. So do not use this wash if your incision still looks deep or shows any sign of infection.

**Massage with oil and herbs.** Once your incision is healed, you can help promote the regrowth of nerve tissue and reduce redness and swelling of the scar with daily applications of St.-John's-wort oil mixed with vitamin E and lavender essential oil. Add one-half ounce of vitamin E oil and three to five drops of lavender essential oil to one ounce of St.-John's-wort oil. Shake well, then put a little on your finger and apply it to the incision with tiny circular motions.

St.-John's-wort helps nerve cells regenerate and can reduce pain, while vitamin E can promote healing and lavender can reduce inflammation. Healing the scar really well could take four or five months, so don't give up.

# Your Breast Advice

They are just two mounds of glandular, fatty, and fibrous tissue located over the pectoralis muscles of the chest. As simple as that sounds, breasts take on a complex role in our lives. They can be a source of identity, pleasure, pain, discomfort, and even anxiety. "If they were just there and not causing any problems, then we wouldn't have to worry about them," says Kathleen Mayzel, M.D., director of the Faulkner Breast Center in Boston. But sometimes, for reasons large and small, we do worry.

The best solution? Take care of your breasts, just as you would look after your teeth, your skin, or any other part of your body. "Women need to get into a regular pattern of breast care," Dr. Mayzel says. That includes annual visits with your doctor for breast exams, regular mammograms if you're over age 40, and monthly breast self-exams.

But it doesn't end there. You should take the initiative to prevent the thing we fear the most: breast cancer. While nothing completely eliminates your risk, you can tilt the odds in your favor.

## Preventing Breast Cancer

In Asian countries, breast cancer rates are lower than those in the United States. Research suggests that the Asian diet, which includes less fat and meat and more soy food than ours does, offers significant protection.

Diet has a considerable effect on breast cancer risk. Here's a list of the breast cancer–fighting dietary changes that you can make today.

**Stay away from alcohol.** The more you drink, the higher your risk of breast cancer. Alcohol seems to interfere with your liver's ability to clear excess estrogen from your body. That's bad. The higher your exposure to estrogen, research finds, the higher your breast cancer risk.

**Buy colorful produce.** Fruits and vegetables are good sources of cancer-fighting vitamin C and beta-carotene. This is particularly true of the bright orange, yellow, red, and green fruits and vegetables, such as butternut squash, oranges, peaches, sweet red peppers, and spinach.

Cabbage, broccoli, brussels sprouts, kale, and collard greens are also rich in phytochemicals (healing chemicals naturally found in plants) that may inhibit estrogen synthesis and guard you against estrogen overload. In one study, women who ate the most fruits and vegetables were least likely to get breast cancer.

**Reach for olive oil.** Because it is mostly made up of monounsaturated fat, olive oil doesn't affect your body the way that saturated fat (found in animal fats and some plant-based fats such as palm and coconut oil) does. A study of more than 2,000 women in Greece suggests that those who used olive oil more than once a day had a 25 percent lowered risk of breast cancer.

**Savor soy foods.** Soybeans, soy nuts, soy milk, and other soy foods are rich in phytoestrogens, plant chemicals that seem to protect against breast cancer. As these compounds latch on to your body's estrogen receptor cells, they crowd out your body's own estrogen, a suspected "fuel" for breast cancer. Women who live in countries where people eat lots of soy have lower rates of breast cancer.

**Eat fatty fish.** Substances known as omega-3 fatty acids are found in fish like tuna and salmon. In the laboratory, mice injected with human breast cancer cells developed smaller, less invasive tumors when fed these fatty acids.

**Toss in flaxseeds.** These tiny edible seeds contain substances called lignans that seem to help fight off breast cancer. Studies at the University of Toronto suggest that flaxseed both inhibits and slows the progression of breast cancer. Grind the seed in a coffee grinder or food processor for a few seconds so that it's easier to digest.

## THE RIGHT WAY TO EXAMINE YOUR BREASTS

To detect breast cancer in its early, most treatable stages, your doctor should examine your breasts once a year during your routine checkup. But your breasts can change in between yearly visits. So it's important to examine your breasts yourself once a month. Also, if you're over 40, you should talk with your doctor about regular mammograms.

A breast self-exam takes only a few minutes. Here's how to do one.

Start by choosing a date for your monthly self-exam. If you're still menstruating, it's best to perform your self-exam after your monthly period, when your breasts are less likely to be tender or swollen, says Margaret Polaneczky, M.D., assistant professor of obstetrics and gynecology at New York Hospital–Cornell Medical Center in New York City. If you no longer menstruate, choose a date that's easy to remember, like the first of each month. Then follow these steps. If you find a lump, discharge, or any other changes in your breast, see your doctor right away.

1. Stand in front of a mirror with your arms at your sides. Visually check both breasts and nipples for anything unusual, such as puckering, dimpling, or scaliness.

2. Place your hands behind your head and press your hands forward. Look for any change in the shape of your breasts.

3. Place your hands on your hips. Push your shoulders and elbows forward and bend toward the mirror. Again, look for any change in the shape of your breasts.

4. Gently squeeze each nipple to check for discharge. Discharge from the white bumps around the nipple, known as Montgomery's glands, is totally normal. A little milk or greenish discharge from the nipple itself is not uncommon in women who have had children or who are taking birth control pills. A bloody or clear discharge from the nipple, however, is cause for concern.

5. Raising one arm, use the fingers of your other hand to feel for any fixed, hard, unusual lumps in your breast and the surrounding area, including the armpit area and

the region below your collarbone. Be sure to cover the entire surface of your breast, using a specific pattern: lines, circles, or wedges. (Some women find it easier to perform this step in the shower when their skin is soapy.) Repeat on your other breast.

**Line Pattern**

**Circular Pattern**

**Wedge Pattern**

6. Repeat step 5 while lying on your back, with one arm over your head and a pillow under your shoulder. This is a position that flattens out the breast, making it easier to feel for lumps.

Then sprinkle the seed on your cereal or salad. Flaxseed oil won't do, though; it doesn't contain enough lignan.

**Cut out the fat.** Population studies show that every country where the diet is low in fat has a low risk of breast cancer, and every country where the diet is high in fat has a high risk. Unfortunately, moderate reductions in fat intake don't seem to help much. Think major cuts.

**Fill up with fiber.** A high-fiber diet may help the body cleanse itself of excess estrogen. It'll also help you control your weight, because bulky high-fiber food fills you up before you can pack in lots of calories. Weight control is key since body fat actually manufactures a type of estrogen.

**Flavor with garlic.** This savory, aromatic herb seems to stimulate the immune system. Garlic appears to protect against a wide variety of cancers, including breast cancer.

**Make green tea.** Asian societies in which women consume a lot of green tea tend to have less breast cancer and less cancer in general. Plant chemicals called polyphenols seem to be responsible. You can also get polyphenols (although in small amounts) in black tea. Look for green tea in your supermarket.

**Get out and exercise.** When researchers at Arizona State University in Tempe analyzed numerous studies, they found that women who pursued very active jobs, such as teaching physical education, could have up to 50 percent less chance of getting breast cancer than those with sedentary jobs, such as doing office work.

Researchers suggest that mod-erate physical activity is a deterrent to breast cancer because exercise helps lower weight and body fat, which means that the body is ex-posed to lower levels of estrogen.

## Fibrocystic Changes

Few things in life are as un-nerving as feeling a lump or pain in your breast. You may be the most unflappable of women, without a hypochondriac's aching bone in your body, yet still find yourself thinking the worst. The good news is, most lumps aren't cancerous, and pain is rarely a sign of breast cancer. Truth is, normal breast tissue feels lumpy and may feel painful at various points during your menstrual cycle.

What's going on? Two condi-tions, fibrocystic breast changes and what doctors call fibroadenoma, are associated with changes in the breast. If you have a fibrocystic con-dition, your breasts will feel both lumpy and painful before your pe-riod. The milk glands in your breasts may enlarge and feel like hard lumps, your breasts' connective tissue may thicken and feel ropy, or the glands may get blocked and filled with fluid, forming cysts.

With a fibroadenoma, your milk glands enlarge, forming a nodule that feels like a solid, rubbery lump. If you have a fibroadenoma, you won't have pain, and the lumpiness won't change over the course of your cycle.

Alternative remedies can help shrink noncancerous lumps and prevent new ones. And various alternatives to pre-scription and over-the-counter painkillers can help relieve breast tenderness and pain and keep lumps at bay. If your breasts become more tender and swollen after a day or two or they still hurt after three months, see your doctor.

**Reduce lumps with evening primrose.** An effective anti-inflammatory, evening prim-rose oil can soothe pain and help shrink lumps. Look for evening primrose oil in health food stores and add a tablespoon to your morning oatmeal or sprinkle it over your salad. Or take one or two capsules two or three times a day.

*Caution:* Don't use evening primrose oil during pregnancy; it may cause miscarriage or premature labor.

**Can colas, tea, and coffee.** Cola, choco-late, tea, and coffee all contain methylxanthines, naturally occurring substances that may con-tribute to lumpiness and pain.

**Brew a cup of herbal tea.** Corn silk and buchu, herbal teas found at health food stores, act as mild diuretics that can flush out some of the fluid that contributes to breast discomfort.

**Up your fiber.** Consume at least 30 grams of fiber a day. Both kinds of fiber, soluble and insoluble, help escort excess estrogen from your body.

**Add vitamin E.** Some studies have shown that vitamin E—when taken in quantities slightly larger than the recommended daily value—is very effective in relieving breast ten-derness and discomfort from fibrocystic breasts. You can start by taking 30 international units (IU) of E a day (that's the recommended daily value amount) and increasing it when you expe-rience breast problems. Or you could simply take 200 to 400 IU of vitamin E every day. But don't take more. Vitamin E is stored in your body fat, so too much could be toxic.

**Soothe with vitamin C.** When pain and lumpiness are at their worst, try 500 milligrams of vitamin C every couple of hours, for a total daily intake of 3,000 to 5,000 milligrams. Doses this high will ease and prevent inflammation. Excess vitamin C may cause diarrhea in some people.

## Sagging Breasts

Legend has it that Marie Antoinette's breasts were so perfectly formed that they served as the inspiration for the classic saucer-shaped cham-pagne glass. Had the French Revolution not inter-vened, though, even her imperious bosom would have bowed eventually—to the force of gravity.

Tissues called ligaments hold up the breasts. Unfortunately, they aren't very strong and can lose elasticity with pregnancy, nursing, and age. Although some of these changes are unavoid-able, there are steps you can take to keep your breasts on the up-and-up.

**Get the right support.** A good support bra allows for minimal bounce and puts less stress on your ligaments. The more you wear one during the day, the more it helps. A sports bra, which adds the strongest support, is especially impor-tant if you jog, play tennis, do aerobics, or par-ticipate in other forms of exercise.

**Push them up.** Not with a bra, but with a pushup exercise. Exercise won't build up breasts that are already sagging, because breast tissue is mostly fat. But this pushup will build up the pectoral muscle underneath, which will make your breasts look perkier.

Lie on your stomach with your hands next to your chest. Straighten your arms and push up your torso, keeping your head aligned with your torso, your back straight, and your knees on the floor. Slowly return to your starting position. Aim for three sets of 12 repetitions each. Rest for 1½ minutes between sets.

**Start to fly.** To build more muscle, try what's called the dumbbell fly, using a pair of one- to three-pound weights.

To start, pick up one weight in each hand, then lie on your back on a carpeted floor or an exercise mat. Extend your arms out on the floor at shoulder level, with your palms up, clutching your weights. The weights should be parallel to your body. Draw both arms straight up together above your body, keeping your elbows slightly bent, so that the weights meet over your chest. Then, return the weights to your sides at shoulder height, as if you were drawing a semicircle or half-moon over your body. Repeat the exercise 12 to 15 times, then rest for 1½ minutes. Do three sets, resting between each set.

The stronger you become, the more weight you'll be able to handle. This means that you should be able to gradually increase the weights you use (by one or two pounds). As you use heavier weights, decrease the number of repetitions you do, aiming for 8 to 10 repetitions per set. Continue to do three sets.

**Rub on sun protection.** Sun exposure can speed up the aging of elastin fibers that keep your skin from sagging. So make sure that you apply sunscreen to your chest area whenever you wear a sundress, tank top, or bathing suit with a low neckline. Many dermatologists recommend a sun protection factor (SPF) of 15. Whatever you use, don't forget to reapply regularly.

## Bra Problems

Some are designed with style in mind, while others purely offer support. But whether it's black silk or no-nonsense white cotton, a bra can make it or break it when it comes to breast support and daily comfort. Bras can chafe, irritate the skin, or let you down when you need support the most—especially if you're large-breasted.

But your bra doesn't have to sentence you to a lifetime of discomfort. By taking a few commonsense steps, you can find comfort and support in this vital undergarment.

**Test-drive your bra.** To make sure that a bra fits, always try it on before you buy it. The cups should completely contain your breasts, with no bulges at the tops or sides of the cups. The bra should be comfortable enough for you to slip a finger under the band at the base of the cups. If there are wrinkles in the cups, it means the bra is too large. Also, make sure that the bra doesn't ride up in the back. If it does, the bra may be too large, or hooked too loosely, or the straps may be too tight.

**Look for comfort.** Check inside the cups and make sure that there are no seams or anything else that may push up against you. If there is an underwire, choose one that is very well-padded so that it doesn't add to the friction.

**Search for thickness.** Large-breasted women should buy bras with thick straps, which support the breasts better and do not cut into the shoulders. For the same effect, you can also buy strap pads and attach them yourself.

**Sport the right bra.** If you're a C cup or larger and in the market for a sports bra, look for one with good support that controls your breast movement. Some women find that nonelastic shoulder straps are best for minimizing movement. Sports bras are available in the lingerie departments of some department stores or in sporting goods stores.

**Rise a size.** Wear a larger-size bra when your breasts hurt. Select one that keeps your breasts secure without being uncomfortably constricting. A sports bra with a wide elastic band may be your best bet.

**Take it off.** If your bra has chafed your skin, ease the irritation by going braless at home. Pull on a peasant dress, caftan, or loose, comfortable shirt that allows air to circulate freely around your breasts.

**Soothe them with calendula cream.** If your breasts are chafed and irritated, smooth on a healing cream made with the herb calendula. Researchers have found that calendula extracts can decrease swelling and increase skin-healing activity. They're antiseptic, too. Look for calendula cream in the health food store.

**Try aloe vera.** Snip a leaf from the easy-to-grow aloe vera plant on your windowsill, slit it open, and scoop out the cool, clear gel that's inside. Smooth it on chafed skin for cooling relief.

## WOMEN ASK WHY

### Why are doctors always warning women not to go braless?

If any doctors have spoken out against the minor "crime" of going braless, it's not in response to a particular health concern. Forgoing the brassiere is by no means dangerous—the bra is simply an ingenious supportive device designed to provide comfort, nothing more.

A concern among many women, however, is that not wearing a bra will lead to sagging breasts later in life. While not a major medical concern, sagging breasts do provoke a little bit of justifiable anxiety.

There's no proof that wearing a bra will keep gravity from taking its toll on your bosom's uplift, but a good support bra may somewhat reduce strain on the ligaments that hold up the breasts. Of course, once breasts have already begun to sag, a bra helps by holding them in the position that we wish they still held.

There is one time in a woman's life when she should wear a bra: during and after pregnancy. Then, a well-fitting support bra will cradle the extra weight of your breasts.

**Expert consulted**
Mary Beth Hasselquist, M.D.
Staff physician
Group Health Cooperative of Puget Sound
Clinical assistant professor
University of Washington
Seattle

# No-Pause Menopause

For a woman, menopause is aging's main event.

Physically, her body undergoes significant changes—her periods come to an end and hormone levels decline, often causing a range of discomforts such as hot flashes and vaginal dryness.

Mentally, she experiences emotional ups and downs that come with surging hormones and the knowledge that the body that she has been familiar with for some 40 years is forever changing.

Spiritually, she faces new possibilities and challenges as she exits her childbearing years for things unknown.

All told, many women say that these multiple changes are a good thing.

"Menopause is positive if you make it positive," says Helen Healy, N.D., a naturopathic physician and owner and director of the Wellspring Naturopathic Clinic in St. Paul, Minnesota. "Many women feel free and glad that they don't have to be concerned with monthly periods anymore."

Officially, you haven't "arrived" at menopause until you've gone one full year without a period. While it's different for every woman, this usually happens sometime after age 50. But you may begin noticing signs of this approaching transition in your early forties—or even in your midthirties.

During this period of very gradual change, called perimenopause, a woman's supply of the female hormone estrogen starts to waver, which can create some of the same problems women get in the throes of menopause—hot flashes, vaginal dryness, mood swings, and sleeping problems. Of course, not everyone has such discomfort: As many as one in three women sail through menopause symptom-free.

The biggest negative of menopause is that it leaves us open to some serious health problems. That's because estrogen is a natural fortress against heart disease, bone loss, and breast cancer. To compensate for the loss of estrogen, many doctors today recommend hormone replacement therapy (HRT).

## Easing into Menopause

Whether to take HRT is a decision you should make in consultation with your doctor.

Sometimes, natural treatments such as herbs, exercise, healing foods, and vitamins can be just as effective as HRT for relieving symptoms of menopause, says Dr. Healy. "If you can do what women did in the past—which was exercise a lot, eat well, and use herbs—you may not even need to take hormones at all," she says. Here are some natural healing ideas for the menopause years.

**Combine some herbs.** An herbal product specifically formulated for menopause may help lessen hormone-related discomforts such as hot flashes and mood swings. Such a product usually contains some combination of the following herbs: chasteberry (sometimes called vitex), black cohosh, dong quai, panax ginseng (sometimes called Asian ginseng), and licorice root.

You will find these herbal blends in health food stores. Look for a product that contains standardized extracts. A standardized extract is guaranteed to contain a specific amount of an herb's active ingredient.

*Note:* Dong quai causes some people to become more sensitive to the sun. So if you choose a product containing this herb, be especially cautious when you head outdoors. Also, if you choose a product containing licorice root, do not use it for more than six weeks and avoid its use if you have diabetes, high blood pressure, or a liver or kidney disorder.

**Eat grazefully.** Eating small meals two to three hours apart may help you avoid menopausal weight gain.

---

## THE NATURAL ROUTE TO HORMONE REPLACEMENT

When the time comes to consider hormone replacement therapy to ease the transition into life's prime time, consider "going natural," says Connie Catellani, M.D., medical director at the Miro Center for Integrative Medicine in Evanston, Illinois.

Choose one of the plant-based progesterone creams available in health food stores. And eat soy foods (such as tofu, flavored soy milk, or roasted soybeans), which are rich in isoflavones, a plant-based form of estrogen.

Studies show that women who eat soy foods regularly have fewer hot flashes. Just one cup of raw soybeans adds about 300 milligrams of isoflavones, about the amount of estrogen you'd get in one tablet of the synthetic estrogen supplement called Premarin. And, says Dr. Catellani, the progesterone in so-called natural progesterone creams (sold under brand names including NatraGest and Pro-Gest) has a molecular structure identical to that of the body's own "homemade" progesterone. The result is fewer side effects.

In contrast, synthetic hormone supplements—sold under brand names including Premarin and Provera—have a molecular "shape" slightly different from that produced by the body. These forms are more potent and last longer and can cause more side effects, Dr. Catellani says.

It's important to note that both natural and synthetic hormone supplements are made in pharmaceutical laboratories from sources including wild yams and soybeans (and, in the case of Premarin, from the urine of pregnant horses). "The natural products are natural because of their structure, not because of their origins," Dr. Catellani notes.

---

**Watch your cholesterol.** Estrogen seems to protect a woman's heart by keeping cholesterol levels in line. After menopause, women have higher levels of artery-clogging low-density lipoprotein (LDL) cholesterol and lower levels of artery-cleaning high-density lipoprotein (HDL) cholesterol.

Studies show that limiting fat to 25 to 30 percent of your daily calories will help keep the bad guys under control.

**Stay active.** Research has proved that regular exercise helps combat weight gain, heart disease, and osteoporosis— problems that a woman is more likely to experience following menopause.

So start walking, swimming, biking, rowing, jogging, or take an aerobics class (or pop an aerobics video into your home VCR). Any activity that elevates your heart rate will help.

**Chat with your partner.** Open communication with your significant other is especially important now. Share your menopausal experiences and thoughts with him, and the two of you will grow closer. It's especially important to address physical changes that can impact shared activities, such as vaginal dryness that can make sex uncomfortable or hot flashes that might leave you a little distracted for a moment at a social gathering.

**Keep your B and C up.** Take 1,000 milligrams of vitamin C and 50 milligrams of B-complex vitamins twice each day. (Make sure that your B-complex supplement contains pantothenic acid.) These vitamins support your adrenal glands, tiny powerhouses on top of your kidneys that continue to produce small amounts of estrogen.

*Note:* Some people experience diarrhea when they take more than 1,000 milligrams of vitamin C a day. If this happens to you, simply reduce your intake of the vitamin until the diarrhea subsides.

**Fill up on fennel.** Eat at least one serving (about a half-cup) of *Umbelliferae* each day. This group of plants—which includes fennel, parsley, and celery—contains phytoestrogens, compounds with estrogen-like activity.

### REAL-LIFE SCENARIO

#### She Wants Natural Relief for Menopause

At 48, Caroline hasn't had a menstrual period for nearly a year. She figures that she must be going through early menopause because her mother went through it at age 45. At first, the hot flashes, headaches, and vaginal dryness weren't too bad. But now these symptoms are getting worse. She has also noticed that she's gaining weight and her breasts often feel very tender. Caroline suspects that her doctor will recommend hormone replacement therapy (HRT), but she's very uncomfortable with that idea. And she believes that her doctor may not be open to offering alternative treatments. Are natural approaches a good choice for her? If so, how can she broach the subject with her gynecologist?

Caroline's early onset of menopause isn't uncommon. Heredity is a factor, and since her mother was an early starter, it stands to reason that Caroline would follow suit. But much has changed since her mother's day.

Today, many gynecologists can prescribe natural remedies to help relieve symptoms. Still, the subject of HRT is bound to come up because conventional medical thinking favors its use, mostly to protect a woman's heart and bones. The downside to HRT is that long-term use has been linked to breast cancer and a dangerous blood-clotting disorder called venous thromboembolism.

## Hot Flashes

Of all the changes heralding menopause, most women agree that the hot flash is the most notorious. Happily, most research into natural remedies for menopause has focused on this symptom.

Starting as a sudden warmth in your face, head, or chest, a hot flash can spread like wildfire in just seconds. Then, as your body tries to cool itself off, you sweat. The kicker to a reddening, drenching, hot flash can be a bout of shivering chills, as your body reacts to your wide-open pores and dampened skin.

Since her symptoms are just starting, Caroline has plenty of time to consider HRT. In the meantime, there are natural remedies that can help her symptoms. The herbs black cohosh, dong quai, and red clover top the list. In addition to herbs, Caroline should eat soy foods as much as possible. And Caroline shouldn't underestimate the power of daily aerobic exercise to ward off the symptoms of menopause.

When it comes time to take hormone therapy, Caroline should consider natural progesterone therapy. This natural therapy, unlike synthetic progesterone, causes virtually no side effects. In fact, it can help stimulate the libido. And unlike estrogen, it offers protection for the breast against cysts and cancer. One popular form of natural therapy that Caroline's doctor might prescribe is the use of the transdermal cream Pro-Gest. It is absorbed into the body simply by rubbing it on the skin.

Before Caroline broaches the subject with her doctor, she should first educate herself on the pros and cons of natural versus synthetic. If she doesn't get a sympathetic ear from her doctor, she should think about seeing someone else.

**Expert consulted**
*Helene Leonetti, M.D.*
*Gynecologist and obstetrician*
*Bethlehem, Pennsylvania*

If you're among the estimated 75 to 85 percent of women who experience hot flashes, alternative practitioners offer these time-tested natural strategies for relief.

**Take a deep breath.** In one study, women who had experienced 20 or more hot flashes a day reduced that number by half with the help of deep breathing.

When you feel a hot flash creeping up on you, prepare for deep breathing by sitting up straight and loosening your belt or waistband if it feels tight. Begin by exhaling through your nose longer than you normally would. Then inhale through your nose slowly and deeply, filling your lungs from the bottom up while keeping your belly relaxed. When your chest is fully expanded, exhale slowly and deeply, as if sighing. Continue until the hot flash subsides.

**Cool with black cohosh.** Black cohosh has been shown to be as effective as estrogen for the relief of hot flashes. You may need to use it for up to four weeks before you feel better, however.

To find the best dosage, start by taking 10 drops of black cohosh tincture (also known as an extract), in a small amount of water or juice twice a day. Then increase the dose by 5 drops every other day until you are satisfied with the results.

Some women take black cohosh daily. Others take it simply when needed. Some women find relief by taking it for two consecutive weeks each month. Experiment to see what works best for you, but don't take it for more than six months, for it could have some side effects such as diarrhea, abdominal pain, and headache.

**Say yes to soy.** Cool hot flashes by consuming 30 to 50 milligrams of isoflavones each day. Isoflavones are plant substances found in abundance in soy foods and supplements. Thanks to their weak estrogen-like effect in the human body, these compounds may help cool hot flashes.

**Start a bath.** Before going to bed, draw a comfortably warm—not hot—bath. Then soak in it long enough for the water to cool, which should take about 20 minutes. This bedtime ritual may interrupt a pattern of night sweats (nocturnal hot flashes) so that they occur less frequently and are less severe.

To enhance the therapeutic effects of your bath, add the following essential oils: 4 drops of chamomile, 6 drops of lemon, and 10 drops of evening primrose. Chamomile is said to relax the body, while lemon cools and destresses and evening primrose aids hormonal balance. You can buy essential oils in health food stores.

**Adjust your thermostat.** If you can, adjust the temperature of the room you are in to 60°F. Simplistic as it may seem, turning down the heat or cranking up the air-conditioning is solid advice. Anything that raises body temperature even a tiny bit can aggravate a hot flash.

**Skip hot spices.** Hot tamales or curried chicken may taste great, but such foods tend to trigger hot flashes.

**Cut back on caffeine.** Caffeine is a stimulant and can trigger hot flashes by raising your blood pressure and heart rate.

**Sip some ice water.** Minimize the inconvenience of nighttime hot flashes by keeping a carafe of ice water on your night table.

**Dress in layers.** Stay comfortable by slipping off clothes as your body temperature rises.

## Vaginal Dryness

As estrogen levels dwindle, the lining of your vagina may become drier, thinner, and less flexible. You may notice such changes most during sex—you're aroused, but you're not as lushly lubricated as you used to be. As a result, sexual intercourse can be painful, or even impossible.

While vaginal dryness poses no serious threat to your health, it can be a barrier to intimacy. Here are some self-care solutions.

**Bring out the sesame oil.** Some women report having great success using sesame oil to relieve vaginal dryness. Soak a Coets (quilted cotton cosmetic square) in sesame oil, squeeze out the excess oil, insert it into the vagina and leave it in overnight. Remove the Coets the next morning, and that night, replace it with a new one also dipped in sesame oil. Repeat every day for a week, then once a week for as long as nec-

essary. The sesame oil may induce an estrogen-like effect.

**Try a homeopathic lubricant.** For menopause-related vaginal dryness, try a vaginal suppository containing vitamin E and a beeswax base. Begin by using one suppository every night for six weeks, then cut back to one suppository one night a week for as long as needed. You can buy vitamin E suppositories in health food stores.

**Chew on licorice root.** Chew two tablets (a total of 380 milligrams) of deglycyrrhizinated licorice root about 30 minutes before each meal. Licorice root targets vaginal dryness in two ways. For starters, the herb stimulates mucous production in your body, even increasing the number of goblet cells (cells that manufacture mucus). Plus, licorice root contains compounds that act as weak forms of estrogen. You can buy chewable tablets of deglycyrrhizinated licorice root in health food stores. ("Deglycyrrhizinated—DGL" means that the compounds in licorice that elevate blood pressure have been removed.)

**Return to the essentials.** If your vagina is parched, you may be deficient in essential fatty acids, oils found in plants and fish that are essential to the health of, among other things, vaginal tissues. Help lubricate your vagina by ingesting a tablespoon of fatty acid–rich flaxseed oil daily.

**Use vitamin E every day.** Take 400 international units (IU) of vitamin E each day. Traditionally, research has paid little attention to the effects of this vitamin on vaginal dryness. But two studies done in the 1940s indicate that vitamin E supplements can improve symptoms of vaginal atrophy. If you decide to try it, give yourself at least four weeks to see results.

**Carry a water bottle.** Drink at least eight eight-ounce glasses of water or fresh juice each day. Even mild dehydration—the kind that is barely noticeable to most people—can dry out mucous membranes in the vagina.

## Mood Swings

It's not clear whether menopause *causes* mood disorders, but it may make existing moodiness more apparent. Some women's emotions seem to be particularly sensitive to hormonal changes at midlife. For them, menopause may unmask mild depression, irritability, memory problems, and even sleep disturbances. Here are some options to control your swinging moods.

**Relax.** In the midst of a bad mood, try a relaxation technique that appeals to you. Some doctors recommend relaxing exercises such as yoga and meditation. Other tactics that may be helpful include deep breathing, visualization, and exercise.

**Soothe with skullcap.** Skullcap herbal tincture (available in health food stores) strengthens the nerves, eases oversensitivity, and helps promote deep, sound sleep. Take four to eight drops of the tincture mornings and evenings in a small glass of water or juice if you're feeling fried, stressed-out, wired, or just wound up. (Do not confuse it with Chinese skullcap, which has entirely different properties.)

**Take a quick walk.** When bad moods occur during low-energy periods, moderate exercise can help. Don't walk so fast that you become exhausted—just fast enough to become energized.

**Eat.** Don't skip meals. As with PMS-related mood swings, missed meals and dieting can affect your moods.

### WOMEN ASK WHY

**Why do women seem to grow shorter as they grow older, but men don't?**

They don't just seem to grow shorter—they really do.

As we age, our bones begin breaking down faster than new bone can be formed. It's common for some women to lose one-half to one inch in height because of normal degenerative changes in the spine. Anything more than that should be cause for concern.

Loss of height is often the first sign of osteoporosis, a condition in which bones get thinner and brittle. While osteoporosis strikes both men and women, it develops a lot faster and at a younger age in women in large part because of the sudden drop in estrogen—a hormone that has protected our bones all our lives—following menopause.

In its early stages, osteoporosis is painless and, outside of a little shrinking, offers no visible signs. In fact, it's usually a broken bone that sends up the red flag. In late stages of the disease, a woman can lose up to four to eight inches of height and develop the classic dowager's hump. By this time, she'll frequently have pain.

Once lost, bone density is difficult to replace—and so osteoporosis is difficult to treat. That's why it's important to prevent it through weight-bearing exercise and a diet that includes plenty of calcium.

*Expert consulted*
*Kendra Zuckerman, M.D.*
*Assistant professor of medicine and associate*
*    director of clinical programs*
*The Osteoporosis and Bone Metabolism*
*    Center at Allegheny University Hospital*
*Philadelphia*

## Bone Protection

Getting enough calcium—from food and supplements—is especially important for women approaching menopause. Without enough calcium, your skeleton can grow weak when estrogen levels fall because this hormone helps bones absorb and retain calcium, the main component of bone. In fact, the highest rate of bone loss occurs in the first five to seven years after menopause.

The good news is that osteoporosis is often preventable. In one study, researchers in the Netherlands found that women who consumed at least 1,000 milligrams of calcium a day—the amount found in about three eight-ounce glasses of milk—were able to reduce bone loss by 43 percent.

Before menopause, aim for 1,000 milligrams of calcium a day. During and after menopause, you need 1,200 to 1,500 milligrams of this important bone-maintaining mineral daily. Try these easy and flavorful ways to get more calcium into your diet.

**Sip low-fat and skim milk.** Don't overlook milk, even if you're trying to cut calories by consuming less fat. Low-fat and skim versions have significantly less fat and calories than whole milk and, glass for glass, provide more calcium because manufacturers replace some of the fat with extra calcium.

**Sprinkle on the cheese.** Just like milk, many cheeses now come in low-fat or fat-free versions. One-half cup of ricotta cheese has 337 milligrams of calcium. One tablespoon of low-fat Parmesan provides almost 70 milligrams of calcium.

**Powder your baked goods.** Add nonfat dry milk to cereal or baked goods, like muffins or cakes. One-half cup of skim milk powder contains almost 420 milligrams of calcium.

**Power up your breakfast.** When making hot cereal such as oatmeal, substitute one cup of low-fat milk for the cooking water, then add one-half cup of milk powder to the finished cereal. This one-two punch delivers 720 milligrams of calcium.

**Pour a glass of OJ.** Dairy isn't the only source of calcium anymore. Many brands of orange juice and other juices have been fortified and have as much calcium as a glass of milk.

**Get a surprise calcium boost—from greens.** Help yourself to kale, broccoli, collards, or turnip greens. These greens contain 36 to 94 milligrams of calcium per cup—enough to help you meet your daily needs.

**Serve up salmon.** Try canned pink salmon *with* the bones. Thanks to the tiny bones, three ounces of the fish contains about 180 milligrams of calcium.

**Take the right supplement.** While food can supply ample amounts of calcium, it's difficult to consume 1,000 to 1,500 milligrams of calcium each and every day from edibles alone. And it's impossible to cram that much calcium into a multivitamin and mineral tablet. So doctors recommend women take a separate calcium supplement.

Which one? Read the label. The best (and least expensive) contain calcium carbonate. These provide the highest percentage of calcium and are well-absorbed when taken with food.

**For enhanced absorption, add vitamin D.** Choose a daily multivitamin or calcium supplement that contains 400 IU of vitamin D, the vitamin that supports bone maintenance by helping your body absorb calcium.

**Maximize magnesium.** This vital mineral helps your bones absorb calcium and converts vitamin D into its active form in your body. Excellent food sources of magnesium include almonds, toasted wheat germ, seafood, low-fat cheeses, broccoli, baked potatoes, and bananas. Aim for 400 milligrams a day, from food plus a magnesium-containing supplement if necessary.

**Exercise against gravity.** Weight-bearing exercises—which include cardiovascular exercises such as walking, running, aerobics, and racquet sports as well as weight lifting—can also help build bone mass. Aim for three or four 30-minute sessions a week.

# PART FOUR

# Our
# Minds

# Master Your Moods

**B**lue Mondays. In a funk. Down in the dumps. Bored to tears.

"Moods are our bodies' barometers as we react to different situations going on around us or within us," says Leah Dickstein, M.D., professor and director of the division of attitudinal and behavioral medicine in the department of psychiatry at the University of Louisville School of Medicine in Kentucky.

Managing your moods can help you get on with your life with your customary energy, determination, and enthusiasm, says Dr. Dickstein.

To achieve your optimal best, here's how you can learn to control your moods—even learn from them.

## Anger

Everyone gets angry. Not everyone goes ballistic, however. And how you react when you are angry determines whether your response is either toxic or constructive to your health and to others.

Think of anger as hot sauce bubbling in a pot on the stove. Put a lid on it, and it will boil over.

Similarly, seething until you boil over can raise your blood pressure or contribute to heart disease. If you throw a tantrum or say things that you will regret, you can alienate others, like your husband, your friends, or your boss.

"Anger is healthy as long as you're not physical and hurt others or yourself," says Dr. Dickstein. The key is learning to express your anger. Here's how.

**Freeze.** The moment you feel your pulse quicken with anger, don't speak or move for a moment. This silent pause gives you time to think about the situation and handle it constructively.

**Inhale the scent of roses.** Take a whiff of rose oil, considered by aromatherapists to be the classic remedy for anger. Place a couple of drops of essential oil of rose on a handkerchief and inhale the scent for one to three minutes. Look for essential oils in health food stores.

**Deal with issues, not personalities.** Don't focus on blaming whoever made you angry. The other person will stop listening and get defensive, blocking a solution. Instead, frame your response with solution-seeking phrases such as "Let's look at the situation a different way." Or

"This doesn't seem fair. What can we do to improve the situation?"

## Bad Moods

Your friends know "the Look." A scowl is chiseled into your face. Your husband and kids stay out of your way. The cat dives for cover. Diagnosis: You are in a bad mood.

Bad moods are more than one emotion rolled into one—usually anger, anxiety, and depression. The following remedies work on more than one emotional layer at a time.

**Walk it off.** A 20- to 30-minute brisk walk, jog, or bike ride—anything that gets your heart pumping and works up a sweat—triggers the release of endorphins, mood-enhancing chemicals produced by the brain.

**Breathe and jot.** Find a quiet spot and take deep, meditative breaths until you feel your heart rate and pulse slow down. Write down what has you in a bad mood. Then take action to undo whatever you did to bring on the bad mood.

"If you're mad at yourself, tell yourself, 'I'm learning something about what I did wrong, and I will try not to let it happen again. It's the best I can do,' " says Dr. Dickstein.

**Grin and share it.** Sometimes, simply smiling at yourself or others can lift you out of a bad mood. So if you are feeling cranky, head for the nearest mirror and give yourself a big smile.

**Sidestep touchy topics or touchy people.** Bad moods can be contagious and spread their irritability and anger quickly. When you are in a bad mood, avoid topics, activities, or people that you know will spark discord.

### WHO'S MOODIER— MEN OR WOMEN?

Females take the rap for being the moodier of the sexes, and it's fueled by the belief that the ups and downs of our hormone levels are linked to the ups and downs of our moods.

While it's true that some women tend to get crankier at a certain time of the month, females by no means take the gold when it comes to the moody blues.

Moodiness actually strikes both genders about equally and has a lot to do with how a person looks at life, says Susan Olson, Ph.D., a clinical psychologist in Seattle.

People who are moody often feel lack of control over their lives, says Dr. Olson. They might assume they are somehow at fault when things don't go well, or they may have the underlying expectation that the world owes them something.

"Moody people can get stuck on a negative thought and generalize it to other things," Dr. Olson adds. "For example, they could say to themselves, 'I didn't do this well. I never do anything right.' "

Gender, however, does seem to have some bearing on how people behave during a mood swing. "In my observation, men are less likely to handle their moods as openly and emotionally as women. Men may appear more angry or withdrawn, whereas many women openly express their feelings of sadness with tears," explains Dr. Olson.

**Turn off the TV.** Vegging in front of the television is the worst way to fend off a bad mood. Staring at the screen prolongs grouchiness and does nothing to improve matters.

## The Blues

A case of the blues is the common cold of emotional health. Instead of sniffling, you weep. Instead of running a fever, you mope. Instead of coughing, you sit in silence.

As with a cold, you could wait out the blues.

Or you could try to conquer them on your own with these remedies.

**Take some B₆.** If the blues seem to stem from premenstrual syndrome (PMS), take 25 to 50 milligrams of vitamin B₆ daily. Two out of three women who try this find that it improves their moods by their next menstrual cycles.

**Strike up the band.** Music lifts your spirits by altering levels of stress hormones in your blood, which in turn slows down your breathing and heart rate. Keep a special stash of mood-elevating CDs on hand to conquer your next blue mood.

**Draw, color, or paint.** If you are upset, drawing or creating anything artistic can lift you out of a bad mood. Keep a stash of crayons and drawing paper handy. Or make a collage out of magazine photos and glue.

## Boredom

Variety is an essential nutrient; it keeps your brain stimulated and your body refreshed and energized, just like a vitamin. Sameness, on the other hand, is like "mental fat"—mental and physical sluggishness that can leave you dissatisfied with yourself or others, unproductive, even angry. Worse, boredom can lead to overeating or bad habits like smoking and drinking. Here are healthier ways to punch up your life.

**Give yourself a new job.** Whenever that "same-old same-old" feeling creeps into your work, it's likely that you're ready for (and need) more challenges. Volunteer for a special assignment or ask your boss for new and different responsibilities. Apply for a new job within your company. Or polish your résumé and look for a job elsewhere.

### WOMAN TO WOMAN
#### She Found the Strength to Heal

*Verna Gates of Birmingham, Alabama, was in her early thirties when a series of devastating personal crises left her emotionally drained and struggling to cope. Spurning her doctor's prescriptions for antidepressants, she instead sought the help of a Native American herbalist. His natural remedies sparked Verna's recovery from depression and changed her life. Here is her story.*

Ten years ago, my world just fell apart. I already had a troubled marriage—my husband was an alcoholic—but I was in denial. I believed that if I kept up appearances, I could survive.

Then all of these awful things happened, one after another. I had a tubal pregnancy and lost my baby, and I got an infection after the surgery that nearly killed me. My husband left me. Two of my grandparents passed away, and my best friend was diagnosed with terminal cancer. To top it all off, a tornado swept through my town and drove a tree through my house, like a pin. I thought, What else can go wrong?

I knew that I had to pull my life back together, but I just couldn't do it. Of everything I had been through, losing the baby was the worst. It was as if we died together. No one else could understand how it felt.

**Tackle a dream.** Nothing stimulates your brain like learning. Make a list of things you always wished you could do—fixing a leaky faucet, speaking a foreign language, painting landscapes, or doing photography. Then call the local community college and enroll in a noncredit class in whatever subject interests you.

**Go from passive to passionate.** Maybe you already have plenty of hobbies, but they are getting a little routine. Ratchet up to the next level. Love to read murder mysteries? Don't just read books. Attend a murder mystery dinner-theater performance, where the audience sorts through clues to find out "whodunit" and why.

My doctor eventually diagnosed me with depression. She wrote me prescription after prescription for antidepressants, including fluoxetine (Prozac). But I was afraid that I'd have to take pills for the rest of my life.

Then a friend of mine persuaded me to visit a Native American herbalist. Chief Two Trees had a little office up in the mountains of North Carolina. He took one look at me and said, "When did you lose the baby?" He had never even met me before.

The chief put me on an herbal regimen that included St.-John's-wort for my depression and burdock root to cleanse my system. He also suggested that I start taking a multivitamin to replenish my body's supply of vitamins and minerals.

I was to follow the chief's "prescription" for 90 days. But after just 30 days, I felt like a new person. I heard myself laughing, and I realized I hadn't done that for a long, long time.

Even after completing the herbal regimen, I continued taking St.-John's-wort for another six months. I still had a lot of physical and mental wounds to heal, and St.-John's-wort gave me the lift I needed.

I still use Chief Two Trees's herbal regimen once in a while, when I feel that I'm not at the top of my game physically or emotionally. It gives me the support I need to get over the rough spots.

**Recruit an adventure buddy.** If your spouse or best friend is equally bored, then tackle adventure together: Put together a 3-D puzzle. Complete a 50-mile bike ride for charity. Join a crew building a house for Habitat for Humanity. No takers? Plunge ahead on your own.

## Depression

If a case of the blues is the common cold of emotional health, depression is the flu. You can't get out of bed. Or you can't sleep. You can't eat. Or you overeat. Or you are sad, empty, or anxious, and it just won't let up.

Mild depression often manifests itself as deeply negative feelings of sorrow, guilt, discouragement, and powerlessness. If you have mild depression, the following home remedies may help. If, however, depression is interfering with your life—if you have trouble concentrating or lose interest in your normal activities—or your depression interferes with your job, see a doctor.

**Pick up some St.-John's-wort.** Fast becoming the herb of choice of Americans with bouts of mild depression, St.-John's-wort supplements work with your body's brain chemistry to elevate mood and ease fatigue without the side effects of prescription medications such as fluoxetine (Prozac).

*Note:* If you are already taking antidepressant medication, take this herb only with your doctor's supervision.

**Turn in your M&Ms.** People who are mildly depressed seem to crave sweets constantly. The refined sugar found in candies and cakes offers a fast mood fix, but the effect is short-lived. Your blood sugar level quickly dives, leaving you feeling down, or in some cases, even more miserable and tired.

Try fighting the sugar blues by eating more foods with complex carbohydrates. Foods like rice cakes, corn on the cob, oatmeal, or English muffins boost your levels of the natural feel-good chemical serotonin and help you relax.

**Seek the sun.** If, like a lot of women, you get depressed and listless during the dark winter months, take a 30-minute walk at daybreak every day, even if it is cold. Increasing your exposure to daylight during the winter months helps you avoid seasonal affective disorder (SAD), a condition that is common in the winter and causes depression, mood, and appetite changes, plus a tendency to withdraw and sleep a lot.

# Best Stress Defense

On any given day, the average woman plays any one of dozens of possible roles: Mother. Daughter. Wife. Employee. Employer. Committee chair. Good neighbor. Volunteer. Cook. Housekeeper. Dog walker. The list goes on.

It all adds up to too much responsibility, too little control, and too little time—the perfect formula for stress overload.

In the world of emotions, stress is the big mama to anxiety, burnout, nervous tension, and worry. Collectively or separately, these emotions can be powerful enemies to the joys we seek in life.

A little stress, of course, is healthy. It can challenge and energize. But too much for too long can pummel your immune system and cause physical symptoms, such as muscle aches, headaches, rapid heartbeat, elevated blood pressure, and irritability.

"Stress is a fact of life. There's no such thing as a life without stress," says psychologist Susan Jeffers, Ph.D., author of *End the Struggle and Dance with Life*. It only becomes a problem when we can't cope with it.

"The best way to cope with stress is to learn how to let go and trust you will handle what-

ever happens in your life," says Dr. Jeffers. "And stop trying to be perfect. Even the Buddha had bad days."

## 10 Natural Stress Busters

Experts like Dr. Jeffers say that it's best to relax *before* you implode. If you're stressed day in and day out, your body actually forgets what it feels like to feel calm. To build resiliency, try the following.

**Take a breather.** Make time for regular relaxation breaks in the day—once or twice a day for 10 minutes.

**Inhale and exhale slowly.** While watching a scary movie scene, you naturally hold your breath or breathe too shallowly. It's an automatic fright reaction by your body's defense system. The same thing happens when you feel anxious.

Keeping this in mind, try to focus first on your breathing the next time you feel tense for any reason. Take slow, deep breaths that come deep inside your diaphragm, located just below your rib cage. To make sure that you're breathing correctly, place your open palm on your diaphragm. Your hand should rise every time you inhale and drop every time you exhale.

As you become accustomed to this breathing pattern, you may want to whisper a word such as *relax* or *calm* as you exhale.

**Conjure up a soothing image.** Picture yourself lounging on a tropical beach or in a hammock under your favorite tree—anything that makes you feel calm and peaceful. Be sure to include all your senses—smells of the ocean or leaves, heat of the sun, coolness of a breeze, taste of a pineapple or lemonade.

**Sweat stress away.** Any activity that gets you moving—such as walking, swimming, tennis, and jogging—generates feel-good brain chemicals known as endorphins while helping to burn off stress-related chemicals like adrenaline, especially if you do them for at least 30 minutes four or five times a week.

**Prioritize your time.** When you find yourself faced with a plateful of tasks, ask yourself, "What's necessary and what's not?" Then do what you must, and let the rest go.

**Cluster tasks.** You may be wasting precious time and not even realize it. For seven days, write down what you are doing every 15 minutes. Review the log at the end of the week. Then try to group errands or delete unnecessary activities.

**Know when to say, "good enough."** Trying to do an A-plus job at every task, no

---

### WOMAN TO WOMAN
#### *She Found Stress Relief at the Gym*

*Robyn Frankel, 38, a criminal defense attorney and single mother from Huntington Woods, Michigan, joined a gym to lose some extra pounds—and was surprised to find that working out brought down her weight and her stress level. Here's how exercise changed her life.*

Joining the gym was the best thing I ever did for myself. My 15-year marriage had just ended, and my weight was at an all-time high. I was carrying 150 pounds on a 5-foot-4-inch frame, and I felt awful no matter what I wore. I knew I had to do something.

When I walked into the gym for the first time, I was so intimidated. I had never exercised in my life. So I started out by walking on the treadmill and now I'm at the point where I run 3½ miles. After about a year and a half, I lost 30 pounds—and I've kept it off. But losing the weight and gaining stamina and self-confidence were just perks. The real hook that kept me coming back was the amazing mental release I felt.

For me, running is a stress release. It may sound corny, but for those 20 or 30 minutes I feel free—like nothing can touch me. It's the only time I don't wear a pager. I don't think about my cases or my kids. My mind wanders. I get lost in it.

Working out is the one thing I do for myself. It lets me take a break from everything that's going on and allows me to refocus. Then when I get back to everything, I feel refreshed. But my routine has to be easy, because if it's not, then it *adds* stress.

At first it was a struggle to fit exercise into to my jam-packed schedule of caring for my kids, arguing court cases, and meeting with clients. But eventually, it became part of my routine. And now it's as much a part of my life as getting up and taking a shower.

---

matter how big or how small, creates a second helping of stress. If you tend to strive for perfectionism, try lowering your expectations a bit. Know when B work is acceptable and give yourself permission to adjust accordingly. Your nerves will thank you.

**Speak up.** Experts say that when you are stressed because you feel powerless over your obligations and responsibilities, speak up.

Faced with too many assignments at work—or too many household chores—you feel overloaded and taxed to the max. So say something. Review your workload with your boss. Let your family know that they're not doing their share. Then divide the work equitably. They may not realize that you're overloaded.

**Take an aromatherapy bath.** To defuse a pressure-filled day, soak in a hot bath sprinkled with essential oils, scents favored by aromatherapists for their stress-busting potential. For stress-induced moodiness or depression, add one to five drops of geranium oil to your bathwater. For an emotional lift, try a few drops of essential oil of sweet orange in your bath.

**Get off the more-better-best treadmill.** All the tension-taming tricks in the world are powerless against stress unless you develop a stress-resilient philosophy. Constant striving for more of anything—money, position, status, possessions, awards, accomplishments—can become addictive and leave you physically and mentally stressed.

To step off this escalator, redefine success. Concentrate on process, not results: Tending a small garden instead of maintaining a big house, reading to your children instead of competing for yet another promotion.

## Anxiety

Anxiety is the emotional phantom of the unknown. It's that vague feeling of dread swirling in the pit of your stomach when you're about to answer the phone in the middle of the night, when your boss says she needs to speak to you, or when your doctor calls you in to follow up on

your mammogram. You're not sure what's about to happen, but you don't expect good news.

If not kept in check, anxiety can raise your blood pressure and heart rate and may trigger stomachaches, restlessness, dizziness, and poor concentration. When anxiety is ongoing or so intense that you can't concentrate, sleep, or enjoy yourself, you need relief. If you suffer from these symptoms, see your doctor.

**Kick in logic.** When anxiety appears, call on logic to come to the rescue. If you catch yourself thinking, "I just don't have the nerve to ask for a raise," stop yourself. Replace that irrational thought with encouraging self-talk such as "I'm a solid worker who has taken extra classes to improve my job skills, and I merit higher pay." Positive self-talk can reduce your anxiety.

**Try some kava kava.** Experts say that this herb is a safe and natural alternative to sedating, addictive prescription drugs such as alprazolam (Xanax). Available in the form of tablets or liquid extracts, kava kava contains kavalactones and, in low doses, relaxes without the sedating side effects of drugs. In higher doses, kava kava actually acts as a mild sedative to help you sleep. For anxiety relief, experts suggest limiting doses to 70 to 210 milligrams of kavalactones daily.

**Take a bath with lavender oil.** To calm anxiety and help you get a good night's sleep, aromatherapists suggest that you add a few drops of lavender into your bath.

**Apply acupressure.** Millions of Chinese rely on acupressure—a variation of acupuncture, without the needles—to relieve stress-related complaints such as anxiety. A quick way to relieve minor anxiety is to apply pressure to the Spirit Gate point, located on the outside of your wrist, below the first crease and in line with your pinkie finger. Press on this spot until you get an aching sensation similar to when you hit your funny bone.

Maintain this pressure for 15 to 30 seconds, then release. For optimum results, do not work the same spot more than two or three times a day.

## Burnout

The math never adds up in your favor. It seems that you have too much to do in too little time, with too few resources—a classic case of burnout. Whether it's involving your job, your home life, or both, the typical symptoms of burnout are the same: exhaustion, insomnia, hopelessness, and an I-don't-care-anymore attitude.

**If you need help, ask for it.** You don't have to be all things to everyone 24 hours a day. When tasks start stacking up, speak up. At home, ask for help from family members or friends. If you're juggling a full-time job with caring for teenage children and elderly parents, ask a friend or relative to step in one afternoon or evening to help you out. Do the same at work and enlist help from others on staff.

**Set aside one hour every day to exercise.** When it comes to remedies for stress, you can't get much more natural than exercise. Working out releases endorphins, natural mood-elevating substances in your brain that dissolve tension. Pick a time—either the morning or after work—that suits you best. Don't let family or job responsibilities interrupt this hour. Select a comfortable, convenient place to exercise—whether it's a fitness center, local park, or even your basement.

**Celebrate small victories.** Instead of waiting for others to encourage you or give you a pat on the back for accomplishing your goals, rely on yourself for rewards. Treat yourself with say, a purchase of a best-seller, a movie, or an iced cappuccino after you meet a deadline.

**Turn off technology.** Thanks to cellular phones, e-mail, voice mail, and laptop computers, you're never out of reach from your office and your work responsibilities. Resist the temptation to routinely contact the office outside regular business hours. Otherwise, you'll be a perpetual slave to the demands of the job, with no downtime.

## Nervous Tension

A nagging, never-goes-away unsettling feeling of unease, nervous tension is first cousin to anxiety. And like anxiety, nervous tension is usually a sign that something you must deal with is bothering you. Outwardly, nervous tension may leave you with a quivering voice, a perspiring face, or shaky hands. Inside your body, this emotion can cause back pain, headaches, stomachaches, and sleepless nights.

Even women who are normally confident and composed can sometimes get rattled when things go wrong. Here's what to do.

**Create an action plan.** The first day back at work after a vacation is prime time for nervous tension. Instead of worrying about how you're going to catch up, get out your calendar. Set priorities. Then systematically attack each item, starting with the most urgent or important.

**Exercise tension away.** This all-purpose tension tamer is made to order for nervous tension. A 30-minute aerobic workout activates endorphins, your brain's feel-good army of chemicals. As the endorphins filter through your body, they provide a sense of well-being and calm. So, when you feel nervous tension seizing control, counter that by doing an activity that you enjoy—perhaps cycling, running, walking, or swimming.

**Shun refined sugar.** If you're like a lot of women, you might be tempted to reach for a cookie or candy bar when nervous tension mounts. Though a sugary treat may appear to be your calming lifeline, its impact is short-lived. Immediately after eating a sugary treat, your blood sugar spikes, making you feel better—temporarily. But within an hour, your blood sugar levels will plummet, along with your mood, making you feel even more drained and anxious. Instead, eat whole-wheat bread or a slice of turkey breast. Complex carbohydrates and protein provide slow but steady energy that keeps you on an even keel.

## Performance Anxiety

You don't have to be an actor to experience performance anxiety. Anyone can experience "stage fright" at home, at work, or at everyday events. You put off calling the new neighbor. You dread being asked to speak at church. You need to make an important business call or have a job interview.

Here's help in mastering your next presentation or talk.

**Prepare—then prepare some more.** If you know your material cold, you're less apt to go blank, and you won't have to spend a lot of time or energy trying to remember it under stressful circumstances.

**Rehearse, rehearse, rehearse.** Keep practicing your role until it feels natural and automatic. That way, when you step up to the podium or walk into the meeting room, you'll feel more confident about being successful in your performance.

**Tell yourself it's okay to be nervous.** A small case of stage jitters before speaking or making a presentation is normal and healthy. Even some veteran actors admit they're a bit anxious before a performance. So you're in good company!

**Visualize a positive outcome.** Cognitive therapy is a quick and easy way to prevent nervous tension from making you assume the worst about a situation. Let's say you're a bundle of nerves about facing your first job interview in years. Instead of convincing yourself that you'll mess up during the interview or that they probably won't like you, inject some positive reality into your thoughts.

Walk into the interview with this thought: "Lots of people are nervous during job interviews. It's natural. She interviews hundreds of nervous applicants, so she's used to it and probably won't hold that against me. And, besides, they called me right after they got my résumé, so there is something about me that interests them."

**Ignore early tremors.** If you start out sounding a little nervous, ignore it. Once you get started, performance anxiety usually subsides.

## Worry

Women, especially mothers, are classic worriers. They can agonize over circumstances that haven't yet occurred or might never occur.

The symptom is a vocabulary with a long list of "What ifs": "What if I miss my deadline? What if I lose my job? What if she misses the plane? What if she can't find her ticket? What if it rains?"

We seem to worry most when we're under stress because stress reduces our ability to reason. But experts say that you can reduce the amount of time you spend fretting.

**Weed out negative thoughts.** When you come right down to it, worry is a bad habit. So, replace the bad habit with a good habit. When you catch yourself beginning phrases with "what if" or "I should have," stop and re-place them with more positive phrases such as "I can."

**Book worry time.** Schedule 20 or 30 minutes each day to brood and wonder. This classic antiworry technique gives you time to explore the "what ifs" and "if only" thoughts filling your head.

Experts advise that it's best to spend this worrying time in a quiet place where you won't be interrupted. When a worrisome thought pops in your head during the day, jot it down and remind yourself to focus on it during your worry time. Try to avoid booking time right before you go to sleep; otherwise, the worry could intrude on your night's rest.

**Consider the worst.** To put your worries in perspective, think through each possible scenario and consider what you would do *if* your worries became a reality. Let's say you worry that you'll lose your job. So, ask yourself, would you also lose your home? Your family? Never find another job? After listing what might happen, identify ways to deal with each of these specific issues. Then let them go.

**Help others.** It's a known fact that the more time you devote to helping others, the less time you spend fretting about your own troubles—real or imagined. Consider volunteering as a reading tutor at a local school, a museum tour guide, or training to run a five-kilometer race to raise money for a good cause. Just make sure that you're taking good care of yourself before you decide to devote more time to others.

## REAL-LIFE SCENARIO
### She's All Things to Everyone but Herself

**Betty is a busy young mother of two with a part-time job and lots of friends who lean on her for advice. She gave up her career when the kids were small to be a wife and mother. And she's never regretted it—until recently. It started after her widowed mother moved in, who relies on Betty to take her everywhere. Every day, the kids' needs get more and more demanding, and it's making her tense and stressed-out. She's bought some stress vitamins containing vitamin $B_6$ to help calm her down, but they're not making her any happier. Short of leaving home, what should she do?**

Betty can take all the vitamins in the world, but they're not going to help her problem. Betty's caught in the web of the sandwich generation: She has become caretaker not only for the next generation but also for the generation that came before her. With a job and a husband besides, it's no wonder that she's stressed.

While a good multivitamin that includes $B_6$ will protect her against deficiencies that may lead to feeling nervous, what she needs most of all is a lifestyle change. She needs to have a good talk with her husband *and* her mom about sharing chores. If she's able, Betty's mom needs to contribute something to the household chores or at least spend time with the children. Companionship between grandparents and grandchildren enriches the lives of all of them. Perhaps she can find activities for her mother at a senior citizen center or with others her own age. She should also look to other parents who can carpool her kids to activities. If she can afford it, she should hire help to free up time for herself.

Betty's feeling stressed because she's being all things to all people, and she needs to realize that devoting time to herself is essential. At the least, she needs to set aside an hour every day for herself to exercise and relax.

*Expert consulted*
*Carol Goldberg, Ph.D.*
*Clinical psychologist*
*President of New York–based Getting Ahead*
*Programs*

# Break Bad Habits

**S**ome sneak up on you like a summer thunderstorm. Others take a lifetime to develop—like lasting friendships. But bad habits—from hair twirling to nail biting, from caffeine "addiction" to reaching automatically for an alcoholic drink at the end of the day—are not friends worth keeping.

What makes these seemingly innocent acts so bad for you? Some can slowly undermine your health. Others detract from your image as a mature woman. Still others can mar your appearance. And let's not forget one other fact: Your bad habits likely get on other people's nerves.

Once you've developed a bad habit, it can be tough to shake—unless you know the practical secrets that can help you replace bad habits with healthy ones.

## A Change for the Better

Regardless of why you picked up a particular habit, experts suggest a three-step approach for uprooting it once and for all.

❧ First, consciously realize you're doing it. Yes, that's *you* with your fingernail in your mouth. That's *you* drumming your fingers on the table at the weekly staff meeting.

❧ Second, determine what caused the bad habit to form in the first place. "If you don't, the chances are slim that you'll stop it, no matter how clever the remedy you try," says Andrea Van Steenhouse, Ph.D., a psychologist in Denver and author of *A Woman's Guide to a Simpler Life*.

Maybe as a child you enjoyed the sound your gum made when you smacked it while chewing. Now that sound is like an old friend you can't part with. Or maybe you turned to that glass of merlot each night as a way to cap off a stressful day. Only now you discover your nightly drinking habit is something you can't break. Ask yourself what need the habit serves.

❧ Third, take care of that underlying need by developing a new, healthy habit.

A word of advice: Be patient with yourself. It may take a few days or even a few weeks to free yourself completely from a bad habit, says Hyla Cass, M.D., assistant clinical professor of psychiatry at the University of California, Los Angeles, School of Medicine. But the results are worth it.

Here are some common nervous habits and expert-endorsed strategies for stopping them.

## Caffeine

Can you remember the first cup of coffee you ever drank? Chances are you didn't instantly fall in love with it. But as the weeks and years passed, you acquired a taste for it. Now, you may find that your relationship with coffee has become an obsession. In fact, you can't seem to function without that first, wake-me-up cup. Or the second. Or the third.

What's going on? Caffeine stimulates the central nervous system, which triggers the release of adrenaline and raises blood sugar levels. As a result, you feel more alert and focused. In the short run, caffeine lessens feelings of fatigue. But in the long run, too much coffee (or any other highly caffeinated beverage, such as diet cola) can lead to a condition called caffeinism (also known as coffee nerves).

The side effects of excess caffeine? You may feel light-headed, fidgety, headachy, or a little nauseated, or experience diarrhea, frequent urination, or insomnia. And that's not all. Too much caffeine may raise cholesterol levels and aggravate high blood pressure problems, premenstrual syndrome, and breast pain. It may put your bones at risk, too.

"Besides possibly raising your cholesterol, caffeine also interferes with your body's absorption of calcium," cautions Judy Marshel, R.D., Ph.D., director of Health Resources in Great Neck, New York. "As women enter their forties and fifties, they need to be taking steps to make sure they are getting adequate levels of calcium to reduce their risk for osteoporosis—not preventing calcium from reaching their bones."

**Take it slow.** You can bid adieu to caffeine successfully if you wean yourself off of it gradually. Give yourself a week to 10 days.

**Stay clear of hidden caffeine.** It may surprise you, but coffee isn't the only caffeine culprit. Chocolate, some iced teas, and sodas (including colas and some noncola soft drinks) also harbor high levels of caffeine.

**Reduce your consumption one-half cup at a time.** If you normally drink four or more sodas or cups of coffee a day, try cutting back by one-half cup every few days. Keep trimming back by one-half cup every few days to allow your body to adjust to the decrease in caffeine.

**Flip-flop with decaffeinated coffee.** After drinking a cup of regular coffee, make your second cup decaffeinated. Keep alternating between the two. Gradually increase the number of decaffeinated cups and reduce the number of caffeinated cups until you are completely "decaffeinated."

**Maintain your "coffee break" time.** If you enjoy midmorning and midafternoon breaks with your colleagues at work, continue this ritual, but simply switch your drink of choice. Fill your coffee cup with caffeine-free drinks such as bottled water, skim milk, or cranberry juice.

**Limit to one.** If you can't completely sever your caffeine ties, drink caffeinated beverages only when you really need to, such as in the morning for a wake-up energizer.

## Alcohol

There's a world of difference between enjoying a drink and needing one—or more.

Drinking too much—which experts say is more than 5 ounces of wine, 12 ounces of beer, or 1½ ounces of liquor in a day—not only can lead to alcohol dependency but also puts you at higher risk for cancers of the breast, stomach, and esophagus. It may contribute to bone loss, raising the risk of osteoporosis. Drinking two or three alcoholic beverages a day also raises your chances of developing high blood pressure by 40 percent, according to a four-year study done at Harvard Medical School. And it can reduce your body's ability to absorb fats and proteins as well as important vitamins and minerals such as folate and thiamin. This, in turn, can have serious effects on the brain, including memory loss, says Dr. Cass.

In the short run, alcoholic beverages, particularly beer and red wine, are notorious for triggering headaches because they dilate blood vessels in your head.

To keep a bad habit from forming into a big problem, here's what to do.

**Get some kudzu.** Kudzu, a vine-sprawling legume, has been used in China for more than 1,300 years to discourage drinking and treat alcoholism. Studies show that two compounds in this herb, daidzein and daidzin, may be responsible for curtailing the desire to drink alcohol. For best results, take up to 100 grams of kudzu in capsule form a day (available in health food stores). Consult your qualified medical herbalist or physician for the right daily dose to meet your needs.

**Try meditation.** If you're looking to wind down, take a pass on the glass of wine and learn meditation. This ancient art of deep, slow breathing helps to calm your body naturally without the need for chemicals.

## Gum Chewing

Maybe as a child you could blow the biggest bubbles on your block. Or you sought to make the loudest smacks with each spit-filled chew. Years later, you chew and smack gum

---

### GOT A, UM, BAD SPEECH HABIT?

It's like you, ah, just can't, um, like, help it.

"Americans are just not comfortable with silence," says Marcia Moore, associate professor of communication studies at the State University of New York in Oswego and a certified speech pathologist. As a result, we feel compelled to bridge conversational lulls with vocal fillers such as "um," "ah," or "like."

Overuse of fillers can divert listeners' attention from your real message, and they can leave the impression that you don't actually have much to say.

You can stop this bad conversation habit by becoming aware of how frequently you really use these fill-in words. Moore recommends the following exercises.

**Record a conversation.** You'll need a friend, a tape recorder, a blank tape, a pencil, and a piece of paper. Record one minute of a casual conversation between the two of you. Then play it back and mark down on a piece of paper each time you hear yourself use a vocal filler. Do this exercise a few times to get a sense of how often you use "ah," "um," or "like." Keeping a tally on paper will make you more sensitive to your use of fillers, and as a result, you'll actually be less likely to use them.

---

with regularity. Why? Maybe because you've grown accustomed to having something to chomp between meals. Or perhaps you fight nervousness and stress with gum-chewing workouts.

What you may not realize is that gum chewing can irritate co-workers and family members. Plus, you don't win many points for professionalism when you look like a grazing cow. Healthwise, if you are chewing lots of gum that's not sugar-free, you may be opening yourself up to dental problems such as cavities. So how can you break this rhythmical jaw-moving habit?

**Suck on mints.** If you like something in your mouth, switch to sugar-free mints. The

**Time your talk.** You'll need a friend and a stopwatch. Again, engage in casual conversation, this time with a stopwatch running. Each time you throw a filler into your conversation, your friend should say "stop." Stop talking for a moment and have her tell you how many seconds of conversation went by before you threw in a filler. Then resume the exercise. Like the first exercise, this one makes you aware of your use of fillers.

**Use a spotter.** A simpler version of these exercises uses just you and a willing friend—no tape recorder or stopwatch. Before you begin a casual conversation, ask your friend to point out each instance in which you use a filler.

**Be silent.** If you're aware that you use vocal fillers, try to stop and be silent between spoken thoughts in conversations instead of linking them with "um" or "ah," adds Moore. Try this a few times a day; you'll build on your success as you find silence easier to maintain than using vocal fillers.

If you want to reduce your dependence on vocal fillers, do these exercises on a regular basis. "You'll probably never eliminate vocal fillers from your conversations entirely," says Moore, "but you will notice a significant change."

taste will satisfy your oral needs, but sucking on these little candies won't result in decayed teeth as marathon gum chewing can.

**Book a time.** Schedule a two-hour time slot each day to chew your favorite brand of gum. Ideally, pick a time when you're apt to be more by yourself, so your chewing won't annoy others, especially if you tend to make smacking noises.

## Hair Twirling

Without realizing it, you automatically roll strands of your hair between your index finger and thumb. Close friends finally confide to you that your habit drives them crazy. Twirling your hair can distract you from stress, but it makes a grown woman look like she's about 10 years old. What's worse, you could lose hair in spots, thanks to the pulling action.

**Find a mirror.** Sometimes, simple bad habits like hair twirling can be curbed by watching yourself do it. If you realize you're starting to twirl, find a mirror and watch yourself in action.

**Reach for a smooth stone.** For some women, hair twirling acts as a way to calm day-to-day anxiety. Try substituting a less-noticeable soothing act, such as rubbing a smooth stone with your fingers. Keep one in your pocket or on your desk. Most folks won't notice your actions.

## Nail Biting

Nibble, nibble, nibble all day long. Every day you vow you'll stop biting your nails, but every day there's a snag or an uneven edge that begs for your toothy manicure.

Experts say nail biting is usually developed out of boredom and as a way to fend off stress. It's a definite habit to break for two reasons. Not only is nail biting itself unappealing but it can also cause finger and nail infections because your mouth harbors germs that are transferred to small tears in the skin around your nails.

**Douse them in olive oil.** Pamper split and cracked nails that beg to be bitten by dipping them daily in olive oil. Let your fingernails soak in a bowl with one-half cup of warmed olive oil for 15 to 30 minutes. Olive oil moisturizes and strengthens your nails naturally. The less brittle your nails, the less apt you are to bite them.

**Keep clippers and files within reach.** If you've snagged a nail while putting on your skirt, shut off the urge to conduct makeshift repairs with your teeth. Stock your bathroom, nightstand, purse, and car with fingernail clippers and emery boards. Keeping these finger tools within reach will help you smooth out the rough edges in a healthier and more attractive way.

**Kill the bite urge with hot-pepper sauce.** Or lemon juice. Or bitters. Anything that sends your taste-buds howling in protest can nip nibbling in the bud. These unappetizing finger dips should be applied daily until your nail-biting days are over—usually within 7 to 10 days. As a precaution, remind yourself not to rub your eyes or the skin near your eyes.

**Reward yourself with a manicure and polish.** Let a professional restore your bitten nails. Select a favorite fingernail polish hue for the finishing touch. "Nail salons are all over the place," says Dr. Van Steenhouse. "That first manicure may help restore pride in your nails. It's a healthy start to stopping nail biting."

## Finger Drumming and Toe Tapping

Maybe you possess a secret dream to be a band conductor. That may explain your need to drum your fingers on a tabletop, jiggle your knee while you sit in meetings, or tap your toes while you stand and wait for a bus. But more likely, boredom and stress account for these fidgety body motions.

Whether you're bored or not, finger drumming and toe tapping can deliver the wrong sig-

---

### REAL-LIFE SCENARIO
#### Her Habit's Too Habit-Forming

Paulette, 42, was recently promoted to office manager at the insurance firm where she has worked for 10 years. She can't sleep at night because of worries about complaints from policy holders, squabbles among the staff, and pressure from her boss to keep things running smoothly. Paulette was taking the anti-anxiety drug alprazolam (Xanax) for a while to settle her nerves, but her doctor cut off her prescription because he was worried she'd become dependent on it. Lately, Paulette has discovered that a few glasses of wine, which she heard is good for the heart, help her relax. Has Paulette found a tension tamer with a healthy bonus, or is she just asking for trouble?

The old saw says "you can't drown your troubles in booze," and it can't ring any truer than in Paulette's case.

Paulette's doctor took her off Xanax, an addictive drug, because she was using it as a crutch. And the same holds true for alcohol. Yes, research shows that a glass or two of wine a day may help protect your heart, but that's not the reason why Paulette is reaching for a drink. As another old saw goes, "she's drinking to forget." What she really needs to do is forget the wine and get to the bottom of what's bugging her.

Because she appears to be dependent on drugs or alcohol

---

nals to others. Even if you don't say a word, your rhythmic tapping could be interpreted as a sign that you don't think what others are saying matters or is important. You won't win many allies this way.

Here's how to stop digits that fidget.

**Join hands.** The next time you feel the urge to tap out a rhythmic beat with your fingers, flash an image of a stop sign in your mind. Rest your hands in your lap, gently holding them together. You'll be more tuned in to what others to deal with her problems, Paulette should consider seeing a therapist to help her cope with her stresses on the job and in her personal life. At the same time, there's plenty she can do for herself to relieve her stress and tension.

On the job, Paulette can make a point of getting away from her desk every hour to stretch, walk around, take deep breaths, and give herself a shoulder massage to release some tension.

What's more, Paulette should be sure to get in some form of aerobic exercise—a great stress releaser—at least three times a week, preferably before her workday begins. Aerobic exercise will boost her spirits and leave her better prepared to handle the stresses of her day.

Paulette also can take some stress-busting herbs such as kava kava, valerian root, and passionflower. These herbs will help her to relax and keep calm before, during, and after stressful situations. She can take kava kava and valerian root right before going to bed as well to ensure a restful night's sleep.

Unlike anti-anxiety prescription drugs, these three herbs are not habit-forming.

**Expert consulted**
*Shiva Barton, N.D.*
*Lead naturopathic physician*
*Wellspace Health Center*
*Cambridge, Massachusetts*

are saying and less apt to annoy them with your finger strumming.

**Watch yourself.** Position yourself so that you can watch your reflection in a mirror or windowpane during a meeting.

**Practice progressive muscle relaxation.** Put your nervous energy or boredom into a healthy, no-sweat body workout. Start by tensing your forehead firmly for 10 seconds. Then release. Inhale and exhale slowly. Move down to your jaw, tensing and relaxing those

muscles, and then to your shoulders. Systematically work your way slowly down to your feet. Remember to slowly inhale and exhale after relaxing each body part. You'll feel more relaxed.

## Teeth Clenching

That clamped-jaw pose may convey toughness on screen for Clint Eastwood, but teeth clenching can wreak Emmy-winning devastation on the enamel of your teeth.

"Pent-up stress is a major cause of teeth grinding and teeth clenching," says Elaine Kuracina, D.M.D., a doctor of dental medicine in Endicott, New York. Here's how to unclench and relax.

**Maintain an air space.** Unless you are chewing or swallowing, your upper and lower teeth should not touch. Make mental notes, or even post little reminders on your refrigerator, bathroom mirror, or near your desk at work, reminding you to keep your lips together and teeth apart during the day.

**Act like an NFL player.** Wide receivers often wear mouth guards to protect their teeth from bone-rattling tackles. The same principle can assist you when you sleep. Try wearing soft plastic mouth guards while you sleep to keep your teeth from connecting. They are inexpensive and available at sporting goods stores.

**Burn off some stress.** Regular aerobic exercise—as little as 20 minutes three times a week—can help you relieve built-up stress and thereby reduce your tendency to clench your teeth.

# Safe Use Guidelines
# for Herbs and Supplements

While taking vitamins, minerals, and herbs is generally safe, experts caution that you should use them responsibly. Foremost, if you are under a doctor's care for any health condition or are taking any medication, don't take any supplement or herb without your doctor's knowledge. Also, if you are pregnant, do not self-treat with any natural remedy without the consent of your obstetrician or midwife. The same goes for nursing mothers, women trying to conceive, and children.

Below are guidelines for remedies in this book that may cause adverse reactions. Such occurrences are rare, but discontinue use if you have an unusual reaction. Also, do not exceed recommended dosages.

By familiarizing yourself with this list, you can enjoy the world of natural healing with confidence.

| Remedy | Safe Use Guidelines and Possible Side Effects |
| --- | --- |
| **Aloe** | Do not use gel externally on any surgical incision because it may delay wound healing. |
| **Arnica** | Do not use on broken skin. |
| **Black cohosh** | Do not use for more than six months. |
| **Black haw** | If you have a history of kidney stones, do not take without medical supervision because it contains oxalates, which can cause kidney stones. |
| **Buchu** | Do not use if you have kidney inflammation. |
| **Cayenne** | May irritate the gastrointestinal tract if taken on an empty stomach. |
| **Chamomile** | May trigger an allergic reaction in people allergic to closely related plants such as ragweed, asters, and chrysanthemums. |
| **Chasteberry** | May counteract the effectiveness of birth control pills. |
| **Comfrey** | For external use only. Do not use on deep or infected wounds because it can promote surface healing too quickly and not allow healing of underlying tissue. |
| **Dong quai** | Do not use while menstruating, spotting, or bleeding heavily since it can increase blood loss. |
| **Echinacea** | Do not use if allergic to closely related plants such as ragweed, asters, and chrysanthemums. Do not use if you have tuberculosis or an autoimmune condition such as lupus or multiple sclerosis because echinacea stimulates the immune system. |
| **Eucalyptus** | Do not use if you have inflammatory disease of the bile ducts or gastrointestinal tract or severe liver disease. |
| **Fennel** | Do not use medicinally for more than six weeks without supervision by a qualified herbalist. |
| **Garlic** | Do not use supplements if you are taking blood thinners because garlic thins the blood and may increase bleeding. Do not use if surgery is anticipated. Do not use if you are taking hypoglycemic drugs. |
| **Ginger** | Dried root or powder used in therapeutic amounts may increase bile secretions in people with gallstones. Fresh ginger is safe when used as a spice. |

| Remedy | Safe Use Guidelines and Possible Side Effects |
|--------|-----------------------------------------------|
| **Ginkgo** | Do not use if you are taking antidepressant MAO inhibitor drugs, aspirin or other non-steroidal anti-inflammatory medications, or blood-thinning medications. In doses higher than 240 milligrams of concentrated extract, it can cause rash, diarrhea, and vomiting. |
| **Ginseng** | Do not use if you have high blood pressure. |
| **Goldenseal** | Do not use if you have high blood pressure. |
| **Hawthorn** | If you have a cardiovascular condition, do not take regularly for more than a few weeks without medical supervision. You may require lower doses of other medications, such as high blood pressure drugs. If you have low blood pressure caused by heart valve problems, do not use without medical supervision. |
| **Horse chestnut** | Can interfere with the action of other drugs, especially blood thinners. Can irritate the gastrointestinal tract. |
| **Kava kava** | Do not take with alcohol or barbiturates. Use caution when driving or operating equipment since this herb is a muscle relaxant. |
| **Licorice** | Do not use if you have diabetes, high blood pressure, liver or kidney disorders, or low potassium levels. Do not use daily for more than four to six weeks because overuse can lead to water retention, high blood pressure caused by potassium loss, and heart and kidney impairment. |
| **Marsh mallow** | May slow the absorption of medications taken at the same time. |
| **Parsley** | If you have kidney disease, do not use therapeutically because it increases urine flow. Safe as a garnish or ingredient in food. |
| **Peppermint** | Ingestion of peppermint essential oil may lead to stomach upset in sensitive individuals. If you have gallbladder or liver disease, do not use without medical supervision. |
| **Sage** | In therapeutic amounts, it can increase the sedative side effects of drugs. Do not use if you have hypoglycemia or are undergoing anticonvulsant therapy. Safe when used as a spice. |
| **St.-John's-wort** | Can cause sensitivity to the sun. Do not use with antidepressants without medical approval. |
| **Shepherd's purse** | If you have a history of kidney stones, do not take without medical supervision because it contains oxalates, which can cause kidney stones. |
| **Turmeric** | Do not use therapeutically if you have high stomach acid, ulcers, gallstones, or bile duct obstruction. Safe for use as a spice. |
| **Valerian** | Do not use with sleep-enhancing or mood-regulating medications because it may intensify their effects. May cause heart palpitations and nervousness in sensitive individuals. If such stimulant action occurs, discontinue use. |
| **Vitamin $B_6$** | Doses above 100 milligrams must be taken under medical supervision because excess $B_6$ may lead to sensory neuropathy, with pain, numbness, and weakness in the limbs. |
| **Vitamin C** | Doses above 1,000 milligrams may cause diarrhea in some people. |
| **Vitamin E** | Although generally sold in doses of 400 IU, one small study showed a possible risk of stroke in dosages higher than 200 IU. Consult with your doctor if you are at high risk for stroke. |
| **Zinc** | Doses above 20 milligrams must be taken under medical supervision to ensure that copper intake stays in balance for proper immune function. |

# Index

Underscored page references indicate boxed text.